BELOW THE BELT

BELOW THE BELT

DENISE WINN

ILLUSTRATED BY MAGGIE LING

An OPTIMA book

©Denise Winn 1987

First published in 1987 by
Macdonald Optima, a division of
Macdonald & Co. (Publishers) Ltd

A BPCC PLC company

British Library Cataloguing in Publication Data

Winn, Denise
    Below the belt : a woman's guide to
    genito-urinary infections.
    1. Genito-urinary infections. 2. Generative
    organs, Female – Infections
    I. Title
    616.6   RC218
    ISBN 0–356–12740–0

Macdonald & Co. (Publishers) Ltd
3rd Floor
Greater London House
Hampstead Road
London NW1 7QX

Photoset by ↗ Tek Art Limited, Croydon, Surrey
Printed and bound in Great Britain by
Hazell Watson & Viney Limited
Member of the BPCC Group
Aylesbury
Bucks

CONTENTS

INTRODUCTION

Most women are likely to suffer from some kind of genito-urinary infection in their lifetime, whether they have an active sex life or not. For some it may be an isolated attack of cystitis or thrush. Others may be plagued by recurrent attacks of herpes or genital warts. Still others may harbour an infection they never even know about because it doesn't produce symptoms – at least, not until undesirable complications occur.

We don't necessarily have to have a 'promiscuous' lifestyle to fall prey to one of these infections. Cystitis, thrush and even the more usually sexually transmitted trichomonas can all be self-generated. Herpes can be transferred to the genitals from a cold sore. To catch scabies or lice, you just need close contact but not necessarily sex. Even the more directly sex-linked diseases, such as gonorrhoea or genital warts, can be caught because of your partner's present or past lifestyle rather than your own.

Whatever the source, these diseases are important because some can have serious consequences if left untreated, particularly for women. These consequences can include infertility, a higher risk of cervical cancer or babies born with severe abnormalities. Other infections may carry no real threat to health, but can cast a real blight on your life and on your relationships

11

if they keep recurring.

Many genital infections appear to be on the increase. This is partly because of the change in sexual mores, partly because of the effects of the accoutrements of modern life, such as chemicals in cosmetic goods and certain contraceptive methods, and partly because there is more awareness of various diseases and their risks, so more people seek treatment, thus upping the statistics. This last reason is all to the good, because so many sexually transmitted diseases which can have serious effects if ignored, respond very easily and quickly to simple treatment.

So it is wise for every woman both to know all she can to aid prevention and also to be able to recognise any signs and symptoms that do seem to signify a need for investigation. That is what this book is all about.

1.
A VOYAGE AROUND THE VAGINA

It is perhaps in keeping with most women's more natural tendency towards tidiness that the female sex organs, unlike the male's, are neatly tucked inside away from view. That does tend to mean, however, that many of us are unclear quite what our sexual organs comprise, where they are and how they fit in with other bits of our bodies. Whereas men carry their all before them, for women the opening to the vagina may be seen as a dark mysterious place leading to goodness knows where. Just as some of us fear that a contact lens can get lost round the back of the eye (it can't), so some women fear that the vagina is a long tunnel down which anything inserted may be swallowed up and never found again. (There are quite a few men who fear that too.)

It is helpful, for this book, to know from the outset what is where and how it works so that we can understand more about what is normal and what is not, why certain vaginal infections and sexually transmitted diseases are more common and why some of them can have the far-reaching effects that they do.

GEOGRAPHY OF THE GENITAL REGION

In her genital region a woman has three openings which are quite close to each other. The first and smallest,

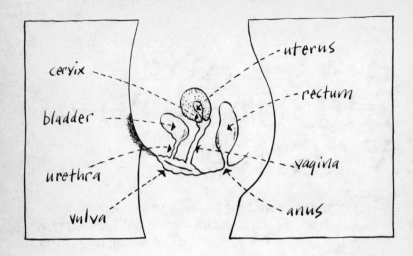

nearest to the front, is the opening to the urethra, down which urine passes from the kidneys. The second is the opening to the vagina and the third, furthest back, is the opening to the anus. This geography itself is much of the reason for many genital infections suffered by women. It is very easy for bacteria, that live quite happily in the anal passage and cause no problems there, to pass across to the vagina or the urethra, where they then make their alien presence felt in no uncertain terms. Thrush, cystitis and an infection called trichomonas can all be caught in this way and more will be said about that, and prevention, in the relevant chapters.

The middle opening, the one to the vagina, is surrounded by two folds of skin, like lips. The outer folds, which are covered by hair, are called the *labia majora* (Latin for larger lips) and the inner ones are called the *labia minora* (smaller lips). The labia minora join, at the end nearest the pubic bone, to form a soft hood of skin underneath which lies the clitoris.

Far from being an endless tunnel, the vagina is only about four inches long and is met, just before the end of it, by the cervix (the neck of the womb). Some women have difficulty feeling their cervix, because of natural minor variations in the length of the vagina or the positioning of the cervix, but it feels a bit like the tip of your nose. It is probably unhelpful to think of the vagina as a tunnel at all, because its walls are in fact collapsible and only open to accommodate whatever is inserted, be it a tampon or a penis.

NORMAL VAGINAL SECRETIONS

The vagina is naturally moist. Quite how moist will vary from individual to individual. Many women mistakenly imagine that they have an abnormal vaginal discharge because they do not expect the vagina to be moist at all except during sex. However, there should always be some degree of moisture and the amount each woman experiences will vary at different times, such as at different stages of her menstrual cycle or because of external factors such as stress.

The normal secretions come from three sources. Firstly, there is a secretion from the cervix which is a transparent alkaline mucus that contains sugars and proteins. Secondly, the vagina secretes a white mucus, which contains shed skin cells and glycogen (a sugar-like substance). This glycogen is converted into lactic acid by benign bacteria called lactobacilli, which live in the vagina. The role of these bacteria is very important, as they help to keep the vagina sufficiently acid to avoid infection (more to be said on that in a moment). Thirdly, another clear mucus comes from the two Bartholin's glands, which are situated on either side of the vagina.

The activity of the cervical and vaginal secretions is very much dictated by the balance of the female sex hormones, oestrogen and progesterone, present at different stages of the menstrual cycle. In the week before ovulation, there are high levels of oestrogen and low

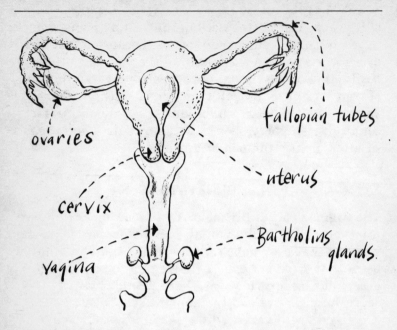

ovaries

fallopian tubes

cervix

uterus

vagina

Bartholins glands.

levels of progesterone, giving rise to a plentiful watery discharge. At ovulation itself, in some women, the increase in cervical mucus is so plentiful that it is called the 'ovulatory cascade'. It may even drench underwear, but it is still perfectly normal. After ovulation, when progesterone levels rise, the rate of secretion falls and the mucus becomes less watery. Just before a period, progesterone levels drop sharply again and the cells on the outer surface of the vagina are shed more heavily, so vaginal secretions also increase, becoming thicker and creamier. During the period, vaginal secretions may be low, which is why some women find it difficult to insert tampons, even though there is blood flow.

Women who use the contraceptive pill may find that they have lower levels of vaginal lubrication but it all depends upon which type of pill they are on. The combined pill, which mimics pregnancy and suppresses ovulation, does not cause any increase in mid-cycle moisture.

When women become pregnant, there is little increase

in discharge from the vagina to start with, but later on both the vagina and cervix step up their secretions. However, pregnant women are just as prone (and sometimes more prone) to certain genital infections, so it isn't wise to dismiss any significant increase in discharge as just a normal part of pregnancy.

During sex – if you are aroused, that is – there is plenty of fluid about. Sexual stimulation spurs the cervix to produce more than the usual amount of mucus and this level can sometimes be maintained for up to 24 hours after sex is over. The Bartholin's glands burst into activity too, as they have the job of lubricating the vagina so that it is ready for sex. Afterwards, of course, all this extra moisture is joined by the seminal fluid ejaculated by your partner.

CHANGES IN VAGINAL SECRETIONS

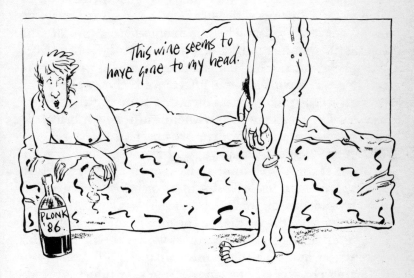

As you can see, vaginal moisture is produced by quite a complex and delicate set of mechanisms. It is not surprising therefore that it can be subject to fluctuation, and not just fluctuation induced by hormonal changes. The normal moisture in the vagina is slightly acid and it is those bacteria mentioned earlier, the lactobacilli, which help to keep it this way. If for some reason the vagina becomes less acidic, certain organisms such as the ones that cause thrush and trichomonas can thrive. Unfortunately antibiotics, especially those designed to kill off a wide range of hostile bacteria, also tend to kill off lots of benign ones too, including the luckless lactobacilli. The result is that the acidity of the vagina falls, which is why many women taking antibiotics end up with a heavy vaginal discharge caused by thrush.

Stress or over-tiredness can also take a toll on natural vaginal secretions, only in these cases the result is vaginal dryness. The reason is that both stress and fatigue reduce the level of circulating oestrogen and the blood flow to the vagina that is necessary for the production of natural secretions. Under such circumstances, sex may be a painful business, because also affected is the part of the nervous system which is supposed to stimulate the Bartholin's glands to produce the necessary lubrication. Anxiety about sex or about your relationship with your partner can have the same effect. As if that weren't enough to cope with on its own, the bruising that can be caused by making love without sufficient lubrication can trigger an attack of thrush or cystitis.

Other things can cause vaginal dryness as well, such as antihistamines, contained in many hayfever remedies, or inappropriate use of antiseptics or other chemicals in and around the vagina.

An abnormal discharge, on the other hand, usually has a distinctive smell or appearance which should help you recognise when all is not well – with the aid of the following chapters. Sometimes it isn't an infection that is the prime cause of the problem, but an oversight like forgetting to remove the last tampon during a period or leaving a diaphragm in for weeks by mistake. All may

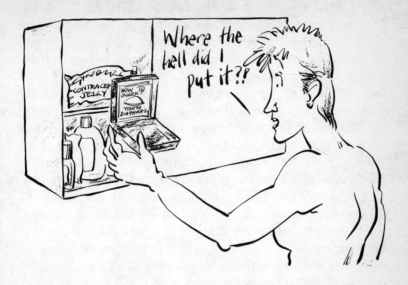

instantly be well after removal but if a secondary infection has set in it can be quickly and simply treated.

There is one more point worth making about the vagina at this stage, before we move on upwards. Because, as explained earlier, the vagina is so close to the urethra and the anal passage, it is quite common during vaginal sex to feel discomfort if you have a full bladder or a fairly full rectum. But one other perhaps more surprising source of pain is low backache, which sometimes has as its only symptom pain in the pelvis during sex. If you have suffered from pelvic pain for which no cause can be found by a gynaecologist, it is worth going to see an osteopath.

INFECTION BEYOND THE VAGINA

Close to the top of the vagina is the cervix, which opens into the uterus or womb. The womb, at its highest and widest point, is only two inches across. It opens on either side into the fallopian or egg tubes, which each run up into an ovary, of which there are two on either side and slightly above the womb. At ovulation, an egg pops out of one of the ovaries and travels down the fallopian tube, where it is available to be fertilised by a sperm. If it is, the fertilised egg then implants itself in the womb.

A number of genital infections can affect the cervix and the fallopian tubes. Herpes can be found on the cervix as well as around the lips of the vagina and can put a baby at risk if present at the time of childbirth. Genital warts also can appear on the cervix, although they are often difficult to detect without a special microscope called a colposcope. Warts spread up the vagina more easily if the vagina is too moist. Herpes and genital warts are both linked with a higher incidence of cervical cancer, although neither is thought to cause it on its own.

The fallopian tubes are at risk of infection from two sexually transmitted diseases, which if unchecked can travel up the vagina and beyond. They are gonorrhoea and one which is even more common in women, though far less well known, called chlamydia. Infection of the fallopian tubes is called salpingitis and can lead to their being blocked – one of the major causes of female infertility. Both gonorrhoea and chlamydia can also cause problems for newborn babies, if they are born while their mother has the infection.

It is a fact, if an unfair one, that such sexually transmitted diseases can have a more dire effect upon the life of women than of men if they aren't caught early. It is also a sad irony that some produce fewer or no easily identifiable symptoms in women, which means that treatment may well be delayed if you aren't first alerted to a problem by your partner's symptoms. So if you are sexually active, whether you have only one partner or many, it makes sense to be sexually aware as well – of pitfalls, problems and, most importantly, precautions. That is what the rest of this book is about.

2.
THRUSH

WHAT IS IT?

Thrush is a yeast-like fungus which is caused by an organism called *Candida albicans*. It is also sometimes known as *monilia*. It lives quite happily in the majority of people's intestines. The closeness of the anus to the vagina in women means, however, that it can quite easily move house, but it can often be present in the vagina without actually making a nuisance of itself. This is because the healthy vagina is normally too acidic for the fungus to establish itself in anything more than small quantities. When, for reasons explained below, it does manage to take a stronger hold, it causes a vaginal infection.

You can get thrush even if you have never had sex in your life. However, having got it, it is possible to pass it on via sex to a man who can then pass it on to another woman or back to you again.

WHAT ARE THE SYMPTOMS IN WOMEN?

Thrush usually causes a significant increase in your normal vaginal discharge. The discharge is thicker and whitish and in some women it is so thick that it is a bit like cottage cheese. It has a strong but not a foul smell.

Your vagina may feel very sore, despite all the discharge, because thrush makes the skin itself dry and there may be little cuts in the skin around the vaginal opening, making it a bit painful to pee.

You are also extremely likely to experience a mild to maddening itchiness all around the opening to the vagina and perhaps even soreness around the anus as well. Unfortunately, for very many women, the itchiness is intense however mildly they actually have thrush because their itchiness is an allergic reaction to the infection itself. Sometimes, however, there is no itching at all and some women do not even notice a particular increase in discharge.

WHAT ARE THE SYMPTOMS IN MEN?

Men are unlikely to 'give themselves' thrush, in the way that women can, because the penis is a much healthier distance away from the anus. They can, however, catch it from a woman partner who has thrush and this is a higher possibility if the man is uncircumcised, as the thrush tends to set up shop under the foreskin of the penis. The only symptom a man is likely to notice is a slight inflammation of the penis under the foreskin and often this is just an allergic reaction to the presence of thrush (just as itching can be in women) rather than a symptom of thrush itself. Very rarely, the thrush may cause symptoms of urethritis in a male – pain when peeing and a slight clearish discharge.

HOW DO YOU GET IT?

Thrush thrives in warm, damp, not too acid conditions and the vagina is not normally its ideal home. Unfortunately, there are a variety of internal and external factors that can change it into one.

First among the culprits come antibiotics. So called

broad spectrum antibiotics are designed to act against a whole range of bacteria rather than against just those causing the particular infection for which you are receiving treatment. Amongst those that get zapped are the innocent lactobacilli, which normally spend their time quietly in the vagina converting a sugary substance called glycogen into lactic acid, which creates the acidic environment that fends off thrush. It takes time, after an attack on them by antibiotics, for the lactobacilli to establish themselves again. Very often, in the interim, the thrush fungus moves in and takes over, making it even harder for the lactobacilli to make a come-back.

Among the many infections antibiotics are used to fight is the bladder infection cystitis (see Chapter 4), which is why so many women find themselves swinging between cystitis and thrush attacks. Even if the antibiotics clear the cystitis, they may precipitate an attack of thrush which, in turn, may creep into the urethra and irritate the healing tissue, causing another bout of cystitis.

Women who are on the contraceptive pill may find themselves more prone to thrush. This is especially likely if there is a highish amount of oestrogen in the pill you are taking, as oestrogen increases the amount of the sugar-like glycogen in the vaginal secretions. Thrush likes sugar. The same is true during pregnancy, when levels of oestrogen are far higher than normal. Pregnant women are particularly prone to infections anyway, because during pregnancy our normal body defences are lowered. If they weren't, we would end up rejecting a foetus because it is, in effect, a 'foreign body'. Unfortunately that means lots of other unwanted foreign bodies can take advantage too.

Contraceptive pills that contain only progestogen (the synthetic form of progesterone) may not be without their problems for some women either. The progestogen only pill (known as POP or the mini pill) works not by suppressing ovulation, but by increasing and thickening the cervical mucus so that it is hostile to sperm. Thrush may not find it hostile, however, as it may mean there is more moisture around.

If the pill isn't the best choice for the recurrent thrush sufferer, the intrauterine device (IUD) is not a happy alternative. IUDs are associated with an increase in genital infections generally. The thread that hangs down from the cervix can act as a ladder for micro-organisms of many kinds to climb. Thrush can very often be a

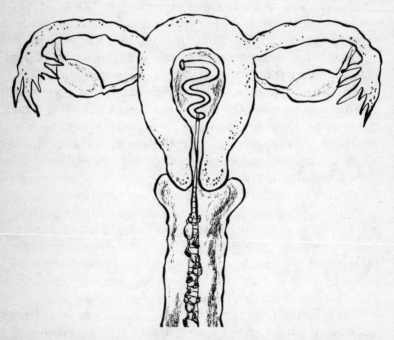

secondary infection that occurs because of the presence of something else. Meanwhile certain women have an allergic thrush reaction to the rubber in their diaphragm and, more rarely, to the spermicides used with it — which covers just about everything except the condom. However, you are unlikely to be highly sensitive to them all.

Regardless of what contraception you use, the time just before a period is when many women find themselves particularly prone to thrush. At this time the vagina is less acid. Some women find that the use of tampons during a period can make matters worse, as tampons have a drying effect.

Sex may be a trigger factor for thrush, particularly if you are low on lubrication and there is rather a lot of friction which generates heat. It can even be your partner's semen that does it, as in some men it is more alkaline than in others.

Because thrush's favourite place is one that is moist and warm, it is very happy with the modern woman who wears tight jeans and/or nylon pants which don't allow air to circulate and absorb moisture. Anything tight around the crotch can cause friction which adds to the problem. Some women like to wear pads in their pants just in case they have any discharge that may stain their underwear. But the pad, rubbing against the top of your legs as you move, can cause friction, heat and irritation, all of which are an invitation to thrush, especially if you tend to be rather prone to it.

Medicated soaps, bubble baths, vaginal deodorants and antiseptics should never be allowed near the vagina, if you are prone to thrush. Such chemicals irritate the tissues and can alter the balance of vaginal secretions. It is also asking for trouble for some women if they wash their underwear in harsh detergents.

Finally, those two popular watchwords of the eighties, stress and diet, both have a part to play in thrush. When we are run down, over-burdened, worried or extremely anxious, our immune system – the body's natural defence against disease – operates under par and we are more open to attack by a predatory fungus like thrush. Poor diet can contribute to our feeling run down. In the case of thrush, it may be particularly relevant, because thrush thrives on sugar and unrefined carbohydrates. Diabetic women suffer from thrush a lot because they have too much sugar in their blood. This leads to increased

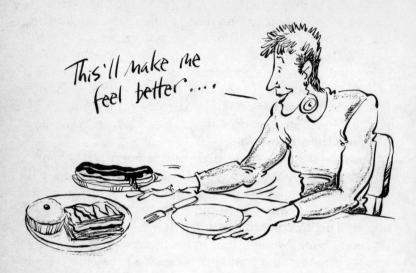

This'll make me feel better....

amounts of glycogen in their vaginal secretions – too much for the lactobacilli to cope with – and increased sugar in the urine which, because of the close proximity of the urethra and vagina openings, also provides fine fare for thrush.

WHAT ARE THE RISKS IF UNTREATED?

Thrush is not a serious infection. However, it can live in other places besides the vagina and generally affect your whole sense of well-being. According to some experts, it can be implicated in some long-term problems such as headaches, heartburn, gastro-intestinal disorders and sore throats, to mention but a few, once it takes firm hold. So, if you do get thrush, it is wise to get it treated.

Thrush may also cause temporary infertility. In one study of 40 women who had no sperm or only inactive sperm in their cervical mucus after post-coital tests, 35 were found to have thrush not only in the vagina, but in their cervical mucus as well. The fungus acted on the mucus making it hostile to sperm, but was eradicated with standard treatment.

WHAT IS THE TREATMENT?

If you are diagnosed as having thrush (and this always needs an internal examination), a doctor will treat you with an antifungal preparation. Usually you will be given, on prescription, antifungal pessaries to insert high into the vagina at night. The most commonly used nowadays are one dose, three dose or six dose pessaries. The one dose pessary is, of course, the most convenient as you only have to make one insertion and you only have to keep off sex for one night. Some doctors feel, however, that it may not be sufficient to deal with considerable thrush, even though the amount of the drug in the pessary is only slightly less than that contained overall in the three dose pessaries. There are doctors who firmly believe that nothing less than six pessaries is sufficient to be sure of success. You may have to judge from your own experience who is right.

If you have itchiness and soreness, you will be given an antifungal cream to use on the skin around the vagina and the anus. It used to be thought that men didn't need to be treated because their penises don't provide the ideal conditions for thrush to survive very long. But current thinking is that men should be given the antifungal cream too.

There are various different antifungal drugs commonly prescribed for thrush, but as they belong to the same general family, all their non-brand names always end in *azole*. You should tell your doctor if you are pregnant or trying to get pregnant, as certain ones are not safe in pregnancy.

If you think you have an attack of thrush just starting, it doesn't hurt to attempt to deal with it yourself by

27

inserting spoonfuls of natural live yoghurt in the vagina – although this can be rather messy and complex! Yoghurt contains lactic acid – the same thing that the lactobacilli convert glycogen into normally in the vagina. Some people swear by this method, while others find it never helps at all. If it doesn't work or symptoms flare up again soon after, do go to a doctor. It is best to see one at a genito-urinary clinic, as they test for everything and have results for you on the spot. Some general practitioners do not examine you and take tests at all, but just prescribe the pessaries on the presumption that you must have thrush. This is not good news. There are other infections that cause vaginal discharge and require different treatment.

Never, if you think you have an attack of thrush, just decide to use up any cream or pessaries you might have had over from last time. You shouldn't, in fact, have any pessaries over because it is important to take the full treatment – otherwise the thrush may just be suppressed for a while but not killed off. The same thing will happen if you later simply use up those leftovers which aren't sufficient in strength to mount a fatal attack on the thrush.

HOW TO HELP YOURSELF

Don't wear trousers that are tight around the crotch and don't wear nylon next to your skin. Cotton underpants are a sensible safeguard and so are one-legged or crotchless tights.

Don't put antiseptics anywhere near your vagina and find some other way to pamper yourself rather than with bubble baths or bath salts. As one consultant gynaecologist eloquently put it: 'Bath salts are just scented washing soda and you wouldn't put that on your face.' Yet the skin around your vagina is even more sensitive.

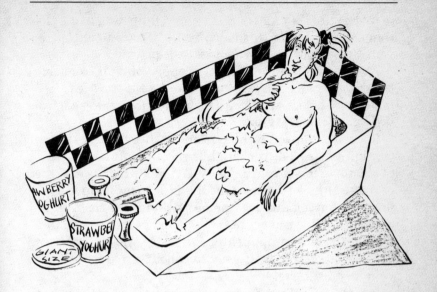

Don't use medicated or scented soaps on your genitals.
Better to stick to pure and simple soaps or, if you can
break the psychological association of soap with
cleanliness, dispense with soap altogether. The vagina
cleans itself and wiping yourself with cotton wool soaked
in tepid water is sufficient contribution on your part.
Another option, especially if you have recurrent itching,
is to wipe yourself with a cotton wool pad soaked in olive
oil. Excessive washing can also bring on problems. If you
have an attack of thrush, dry yourself with a hair dryer
(not too hot) instead of a towel, because that stops you
having to touch the painful area and is also more
hygienic.

There are differing views about the wisdom of baths.
Some say that lying in a bath for a long soak is never
a good idea if you are prone to thrush, and certainly not
while in the throes of an attack as it increases irritation.
But at least one expert claims that nine out of ten women
who suffer abnormal vaginal discharge only shower and
never bath. A quick bath once a week may be a good idea

29

to make sure that nothing nasty is left lurking in crevices that showers fail to flush out. You will need to judge from your own experience which is best for you.

After using the toilet always wipe yourself from front to back, not vice versa. There are various nasties, including thrush, which are just dying for a free ride from the anus to the vagina.

If you are someone who is prone to thrush attacks when you have a period, you might find it helpful to buy a particular kind of vaginal jelly, Aci-gel, which is designed to make the vagina more acid and less promising a prospect for certain organisms, including thrush. It can be bought over the counter in chemists and comes in a tube with its own applicator for ease of insertion. It can be a good preventive if used for about three days before your period starts.

Inserting yoghurt in the vagina in the same way may be equally effective. Even if you have tried yoghurt to

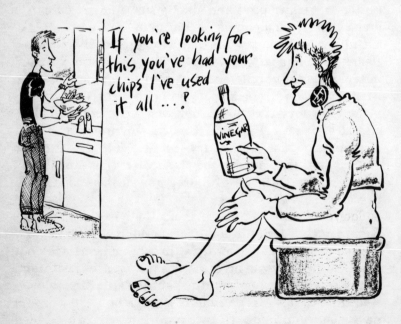

cure thrush and failed, using it as a preventive, simply to increase the acidity of the vagina, may be more successful. Or you might try putting a little vinegar in a large bowl of warm water and sitting in it for a few minutes.

When you have a period, don't use a larger than necessary tampon in the seemingly logical expectation that you won't have to change it so often. Some women find that using tampons at all can trigger thrush, because they are drying. Using extra large tampons is especially drying. For good hygiene, tampons should always be changed every four to six hours, whatever their size.

Having sex when you are not lubricating properly is often an invitation for thrush. If you are dry because you don't want sex, then don't have it. If you are dry because it is that time of the month or you are under stress but you are still feeling sexy, use a vaginal lubricant. There are a selection you can buy in chemists. You can also safely use something like baby oil but *not* a product that is full of counter-productive chemicals!

Some women like their anal passage to be stimulated during sex. Fair enough, as long as your partner does not use the same finger to stimulate you vaginally after. Similarly, if you happen to like anal sex (not highly recommended since the advent of AIDS), do not follow this up with vaginal sex before your partner has had a good wash.

Choose your contraception with care as well. The pill, the IUD, the diaphragm and spermicides can all trigger thrush, but it is unlikely that every one of them will do so for you.

Try to avoid unnecessary courses of antibiotics. A lot of people go off to the doctor with a bad cold or sore throat and beg to be given something that will make it better. To keep the peace, very many doctors will duly oblige with good old antibiotics, even though they have no effect on simple colds and sore throats, which are caused by viruses not bacteria. You are better off sitting it out and suffering, than encouraging a potential bout of thrush for no worthwhile reason.

As a regular thing, do make sure your diet contains plenty of fruit and vegetables. Vitamin C helps buck up the body's immune system and so do the B complex of vitamins, found variously in foods like wheatgerm, nuts, beans, eggs, milk, green vegetables, wholemeal bread, wholemeal pasta, oats, meat and fish. If thrush is a recurrent nuisance for you, try avoiding all foods and drinks high in sugar (and that may mean watching the alcohol too) or refined carbohydrates like white bread and flour.

If you do get an attack of thrush, seek treatment early and ask for your partner, if you have one, to receive treatment too. Some doctors don't think of it. Others still may not even believe it is necessary, even when it is.

3.
GARDNERELLA

WHAT IS IT?

Gardnerella is an organism with a number of similarities to thrush, except that it is a bacterium (a microscopic single-celled organism) not a fungus. It is either as common, more common or nearly as common as thrush in women who receive treatment for vaginal infections in various genito-urinary clinics, but is likely to be under diagnosed by general practitioners. Many people have never even heard of it, partly as a result of some lack of professional consensus as to its name.

It is referred to by some as non-specific vaginitis, which sounds grand but actually means inflammation of the vagina due to something that can't be specified. The term is in fact incorrect, nebulous as it is, because one thing gardnerella does not cause is inflammation. It may also come under the umbrella term of non-specific bacterial infection, but that isn't much liked by those who have made a study of it, as the relevant bacteria can be isolated in tests and are therefore very specific indeed.

Those who did decide to give it a proper name first decided on *Haemophilus vaginalis* and then *Corynebacterium vaginalis*. It was finally rewarded with the much prettier name of gardnerella after an American, Dr Gardner, who had made a full study and description of its syndrome. Even this, however, may not be the end of the story. It is now thought that gardnerella alone does not cause the following symptoms, but rather gardnerella and mixed anaerobic bacteria (anaerobic bacteria live without air – gardnerella can live with or without it). It has therefore been suggested that anaerobic vaginosis might be a more appropriate term than any that have gone before.

Gardnerella is the simplest name, however, so I shall carry on using it here. But it is worth knowing of all the others, in case you are ever told that one of them is your diagnosis. Gardnerella can be sexually transmitted but this is not the usual way to get it – although it isn't known to be found in people who aren't sexually active. In a large number of women who are sexually active it lives quite quietly and happily in the vagina without presenting any problem while the bacteria are in small numbers.

WHAT ARE THE SYMPTOMS IN WOMEN?

Gardnerella doesn't always produce symptoms but when it does it gives rise to a thin, fishy-smelling, whitish-grey

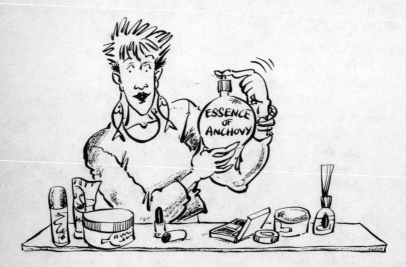

discharge that is often frothy. The discharge may be a lot or a little and the smell may be strongest when a period ends or after sex. Unlike thrush, it is not usually accompanied by itching unless it has been present profusely for some time and caused some degree of soreness. Sometimes women give themselves the itch by trying to use inappropriate creams or ointments from chemists in an attempt to soothe the soreness or by putting perfumes of some description on themselves or in the bath to mask the smell. That is obviously not a good idea, but it isn't always done as a result of ignorance or negligence. Many women are told by doctors who test only for more well-known genital infections, that there is nothing wrong with them.

WHAT ARE THE SYMPTOMS IN MEN?

Gardnerella can infect the urethra in men but nine out of ten men found by laboratory tests to be harbouring gardnerella do not have any symptoms and it doesn't seem to cause them any problems at all. However, gardnerella can be found in a small proportion of women whose partners have NSU (non-specific urethritis, which causes inflammation and discharge) so it may be associated with NSU in some cases.

HOW DO YOU GET IT?

Gardnerella likes conditions that are not too acidic, so the same sorts of circumstances which serve to lessen vaginal acidity and cause thrush can alternatively cause gardnerella to take hold. So treatment for some other infection with antibiotics, which kill off the acid-producing lactobacilli in the vagina (see Chapter 2) but which don't always succeed in killing gardnerella, may create a breeding ground. It often pops up just before a period, when the vagina is temporarily less acid. It is rare, however, for gardnerella and thrush to occur together.

Gardnerella can be caught during sex with a man who is carrying it. It also seems to be triggered in some women after childbirth or gynaecological surgery. And the IUD can be a culprit, associated as it is with an increase in genital infections generally.

Gardnerella can often be a secondary infection. About a third of the women who have gonorrhoea also have gardnerella, although that is not to say that women who have gardnerella also usually have gonorrhoea, because they don't. It is very often present too in women who have trichomonas or genital warts.

WHAT ARE THE RISKS IF UNTREATED?

Gardnerella is unpleasant but unlikely to be a precursor of anything awful. In some instances anaerobic bacteria have been found in association with pelvic inflammatory disease (PID, see Chapter 6) and it is certainly possible that the insertion of an IUD or surgery for abortion could enable such bacteria to make their way up into the fallopian tubes. But gardnerella is unlikely to *cause* PID and is more likely, in such cases, to be just an associated nuisance.

WHAT IS THE TREATMENT?

If you are diagnosed as suffering from gardnerella by a doctor, the usual treatment is five days of 400mg tablets of a drug called metronidazole, taken twice a day or, more recently accepted as equally effective in most cases, one oral dose of 2g.

Metronidazole (perhaps better known in one of its brand name versions of Flagyl) is not strictly an antibiotic. It is an antiprotozoan – protozoa are large single-celled organisms – but it also acts against some bacteria and is more effective against gardnerella in the short-term than most antibiotics alone. However, the relapse rate, as with thrush, is high, though whether these are true relapses or reinfection is impossible to know. Certainly between 10 and 40 per cent of women treated for gardnerella get it again at some time and some researchers are investigating the effects of a combination of drugs to deal with it more effectively. Meanwhile, some doctors think the solution is to prescribe the 2g dose of metronidazole as a preventive, to be taken on the third day of every period, for women who suffer very regular recurrences.

Another approach that is looking good, after trials in several countries, is treatment with the Metro Sponge, which is the contraceptive sponge (marketed here as Today) impregnated with metronidazole. Because the treatment is local, only one tenth of the usual oral dose of the drug is required. Preliminary trial results showed a cure rate of 96 per cent for women who used Metro Sponges, each being left in the vagina for 24 hours, on three consecutive days. If these results continue and a licence to manufacture is granted, this treatment should be available on prescription.

Metronidazole causes alarm bells to ring for some people because it can kill off white blood cells. But you would need to be taking huge doses for the white blood cells to be affected. It should not, however, be taken in the first three months of pregnancy. In later pregnancy, it is given vaginally, not orally.

You shouldn't drink alcohol when taking the drug. Alcohol reduces its effectiveness and also, in many people, interacts in a way that makes them feel violently ill. To do least harm and most good, leave the drink alone and always take the drug with food or milk, not on an empty stomach. Your partner should normally be treated too, regardless of the fact he has no symptoms, although not all experts agree on this.

HOW TO HELP YOURSELF

If you are prone to gardnerella, perhaps before a period, the therapeutic vaginal jelly, Aci-gel (available from chemists, see Chapter 2) inserted in the vagina for about three days prior to a period can help prevent an attack, as it makes the vagina more acid and less appealing to gardnerella. A short sit in mildly vinegared water can help in a similar way.

Some people say garlic works wonders if, at the first signs of an attack, half a clove, wrapped in a small strip of gauze if you like, is inserted into the vagina overnight. Repeat nightly, with a fresh clove for about a week. Unfortunately, there will be a strong smell of garlic and it will not confine itself to your vagina. You tend to be able to smell it on the skin generally, so this might not be an attractive self-help remedy. If you are plagued with repeated gardnerella attacks, however, you could experiment with garlic pills taken orally (available from health food shops and chemists). There are some that promise no smell!

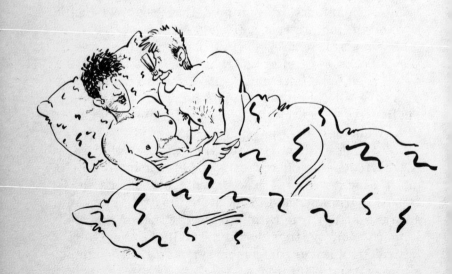

4.
CYSTITIS

WHAT IS IT?

Cystitis is an agonising inflammation of the bladder, which affects four out of five women at some time during their lives. Such inflammation isn't exclusive to women, but they suffer so much more than men because the urethra, which leads to the bladder, is much closer to the anus in women and because the urethra itself is much shorter (3.5cm against men's 20cm), so infections can quickly climb it. The close proximity of the vagina is a source of infection too.

In very many women, the inflammation which causes the pain may be present only in the urethra (urethritis), while the bladder itself appears normal. As conventional examination by a doctor shows only the bladder, the diagnosis may be missed.

Cystitis is not a sexually transmitted disease and cannot be passed to or from a partner. But sex can bring problems of its own, which will be dealt with below, and thus has a part to play in the problem.

WHAT ARE THE SYMPTOMS IN WOMEN?

All sorts of urinary problems and their related symptoms tend to get lumped together under the umbrella term of cystitis. True cystitis has specific symptoms, however. It causes an increased, sometimes uncontrollable, need to pee at very frequent intervals and a burning pain when you do, because the urine is very acid. It is agony when it makes contact with bruised tissue around the urethral opening. Sometimes cystitis can be mistaken for genital herpes, which also causes burning when urine comes in contact with the damaged tissue of an open herpes lesion. Very often with cystitis there is blood in the urine. The feeling of an intense need to pee can occur even when there is nothing left in the bladder and makes many women terrified to leave the toilet seat.

WHAT ARE THE SYMPTOMS IN MEN?

The term cystitis is never used for men, although the symptoms are similar. They are more likely to be diagnosed with urethritis or prostatitis (inflammation of the prostate gland). As there is no relationship between

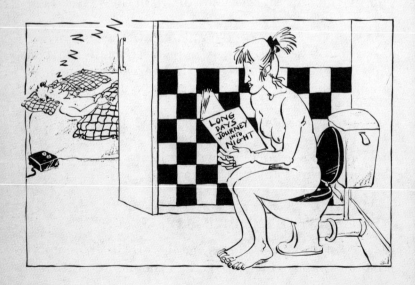

the incidence in men and women, we need not be concerned with the male version here.

HOW DO YOU GET IT?

Cystitis is caused either by infection or bruising or it can be an allergic reaction to certain chemicals.

Infection is very commonly caused by the migration of bacteria called E. coli (*Esterichia coliform*) from their normal home, the bowel, to the urethra. As the two openings are so close, the transfer can occur because of poor hygiene or when a woman has a bad attack of diarrhoea. Bacteria can also pass from the vagina to the urethra if your partner has gonorrhoea or a non-specific genital infection, so besides catching the disease, you may also trigger cystitis.

Sex can also precipitate an attack of cystitis because of bruising, particularly if you are dry. Not only is sex uncomfortable in such circumstances, but the area around the opening to the vagina and urethra can get quite battered and bruised. This source of cystitis used to be called honeymoon cystitis, because women experiencing sex for the first time, perhaps repeatedly at short intervals and perhaps being somewhat dry out of nerves or fear, commonly had their first episode of cystitis shortly after. However, it is just as common in women who are sexually experienced. Often, making love when your bladder or your bowels could do with emptying leads more readily to bruising, as both can be pressed against and banged about during sex.

Some women may have an allergic inflammatory reaction to spermicidal contraceptive foams and creams which gives rise to symptoms of cystitis. Others react to perfumed soaps or to coloured dyes in underwear and to the detergents in which they are washed. The rim of a badly fitting diaphragm can sometimes irritate or bruise the urethra too.

Women who are pregnant often experience an increased need to pee and may have cystitis-like symptoms, but usually these are caused by the pressure of the baby's head on the bladder and not by an infection. However, if you are prone to cystitis and pregnant, you are quite likely to suffer recurrences, because during pregnancy our normal body defences against infections are lowered. Women who have gone through the menopause may also be more prone to cystitis attacks because of the drop in oestrogen levels, which reduces vaginal secretions leaving tissues more susceptible to dryness and cracking.

The onset of diabetes can cause discomfort in the urethra and an increased need to urinate, but not necessarily with pain. Finally, childhood kidney problems can predispose you to cystitis attacks in adult life.

WHAT ARE THE RISKS IF UNTREATED?

A serious unchecked attack of cystitis that is caused by infection can progress to infect the kidneys as well as the bladder and cause pyelitis, also known as pyelonephritis. The symptoms are fever, abdominal pain, sometimes nausea and generally feeling awful. If that is not checked either, the kidneys may be seriously impaired.

The other risk is a ruined relationship. Many founder as a result of the constant agony a woman experiences during sex and the emotional tension that ensues and permeates the whole of the rest of a couple's life together. Recurrent cystitis is no joke.

WHAT IS THE TREATMENT?

First-line medical treatment is usually with antibiotics, if the cystitis has been caused by an infection. A specimen of mid-stream urine needs to be tested first, to ascertain

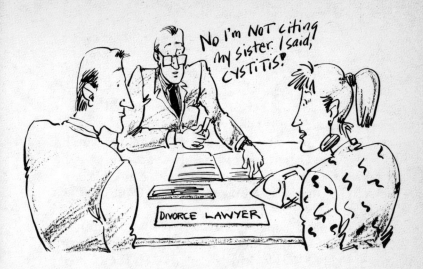

the source. The urine tested needs to be mid-stream because the first drops that come out will be contaminated by bacteria or whatever else is hanging around outside the urethra. There is a whole range of antibiotics that comes into play in the treatment of urinary problems. Which one is prescribed should depend on the cause of the infection and your own individual history.

In some puzzling cases of recurrent cystitis, further investigation may be thought advisable, such as specific X-rays or scrutiny of your urethra and bladder with a special microscope while you are under general anaesthetic. However, much recurrent cystitis can be prevented by the self-help remedies listed below. Cystitis not caused by infection can often be eliminated altogether by self-help means.

If you have cystitis symptoms after having sex for the first time with a new boyfriend, it is worth going to a genito-urinary clinic to be checked for the presence of any other genital infection which may have triggered your cystitis. As mentioned earlier, too, in some cases herpes may be the problem, not cystitis at all.

43

HOW TO HELP YOURSELF

Firstly, anyone who is regularly plagued by cystitis attacks should buy the cystitis sufferer's bible, *Understanding Cystitis*, by Angela Kilmartin. A one-time sufferer herself, she has done more than anyone else to get cystitis treated seriously and sympathetically and to provide a full preventive guide.

Always wipe from front to back whenever you have a pee or a bowel movement and always wash your hands afterwards. Avoid anything, including any sexual activity, which may transfer bacteria from the back passage to the urethra.

Always pass urine before and within 15 minutes after having sex. Wash yourself afterwards. In this way you can get rid of any lurking germs before they hit base. Use a vaginal lubricant – one designed for the purpose as sold in chemists – if you are dry before starting sex. But if your skin does feel a bit hot and sore afterwards around the vagina, cool it down with cold water before washing. It would be a welcome gesture on your partner's part if he would quickly wash his penis before having sex with you.

Drink plenty of water every day to dilute urine and keep the urethra flushed through. This may be especially important before or after a period when attacks of cystitis are common. Coffee, tea and alcohol can irritate the urethra for many women (as can spicy foods). Always have a pee as soon as is practically possible when you feel you want one. Storing up urine is also storing up problems for yourself.

Avoid all irritant chemicals such as perfumed or medicated soaps, vaginal deodorants (never a good idea) or harsh detergents for washing underwear. Wash pants in simple soap by hand or boil them in plain water. Wear cotton pants because nylon does not allow air to circulate, so the skin gets clammy and bacteria can breed. Be aware if coloured dyes even in cotton pants cause you trouble.

Some women say they react to the dye in coloured toilet paper.

HOW TO DEAL WITH A CYSTITIS ATTACK

Angela Kilmartin's method for aborting an attack of cystitis in three hours is as follows. Immediately you feel an attack coming on, drink a pint of cold water. This will help dilute the acidity of your urine and make it less painful to pee. Then mix up one teaspoonful of bicarbonate of soda in a quarter of a glassful of diluted orange squash (not concentrated juice) and drink that too. Bicarbonate of soda is alkaline. Repeat the bicarbonate three times in the next three hours (but not more often).

Also, each hour, have a cup of strong black coffee. This will irritate the bladder, not desirable when you don't have cystitis but useful when you do, as it will act as a diuretic and an irritant of the bladder that will speed the need to pass urine and flush out the infecting bacteria.

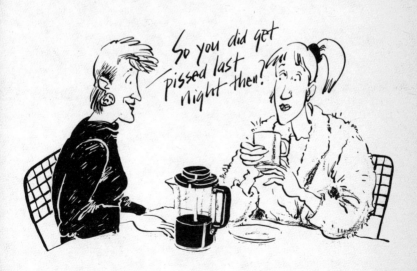

Throughout, keep drinking a half pint of liquid, such as weak tea or diluted fruit squash, every 20 minutes and swab gently around your urethra with moist cotton wool each time you pee.

Take two painkillers at the start, if you need them, and lie down with two hot water bottles, one behind your back and the other wrapped in a towel between your legs, so that it is in soothing contact with the opening to the urethra.

A less aggressive alternative may be provided by the use of Cymalon, which is available from chemists. It contains sachets of granules which should be taken in a drink every eight hours for 48 hours. The granules make the urine less acid and also act as a diuretic.

Whatever method you use, if your urine is cloudy or bloody after the course is over or you have a fever, pain in your back or abdomen or an abnormal vaginal discharge, see your doctor.

5.
TRICHOMONAS

WHAT IS IT?

Trichomonas is a protozoan, a large single-celled
organism – large, that is, in comparison with bacteria
though neither can be seen without a microscope. It can
live in the rectum of men and women without causing
problems. It can also live in the vagina, urethra and
bladder in women and in the urethra and prostate in men,
and then often does cause problems – although less so
in men. When it makes itself felt in the vagina, the
ensuing infection is called trichomoniasis. It is usually
sexually transmitted, but this is not always the case.
Trichomonas is extremely common. One in five women
is likely to get it at some time in her life.

WHAT ARE THE SYMPTOMS IN WOMEN?

Trichomonas doesn't always cause a discharge, but it
usually does. The discharge is thin, frothy, yellow-green
in colour and very often itchy. It smells rather fishy and
pretty disgusting. Because the discharge is itself an
irritant, it makes the skin around the vagina sore and
inflamed and then peeing can be painful. Beware being
diagnosed as having cystitis instead by a doctor who
doesn't do an internal examination and take swabs.

However, trichomonas can spread to the urethra and cause cystitis too. Trichomonas often occurs with other genital infections (see below) and then the discharge may be thick and whitish. Having sex once you have contracted it will probably be too painful, but if you do, you may notice some bleeding afterwards.

WHAT ARE THE SYMPTOMS IN MEN?

Men very often have no symptoms at all and therefore don't know they have got it – or that they are passing it on. If they do have symptoms, these are likely to be a thin whitish discharge from the urethra and maybe some pain when they pee as well. If the trichomonas infects the prostate, they may find that they are wanting to pee more often than usual. There might be a little bit of blood in the semen but you and he are unlikely to know that it is his if you have sex.

HOW DO YOU GET IT?

In most cases trichomonas is sexually transmitted. If a man has sex with you within a week of having sex with someone else who has trichomonas, you are at your highest risk of catching it. It is thought that trichomonas doesn't really like the male urethra and is probably eliminated in his urine in a week or so, if he doesn't in the interim have sex with a woman who can offer a nice, warm, wet vagina as a better home. Trichomonas likes it warm and wet. However, although it shows up in only about 10 per cent of men given just urethral tests, it is found to be present in the prostate fluid and semen of up to 90 per cent of the male partners of women who have trichomonas. So it should never be assumed that your male partner is clear unless he is treated anyway.

Trichomonas is a common companion of gonorrhoea – about 40 per cent of women suffering the latter also have the former. At a genito-urinary clinic, if you have symptoms of trichomonas, you will always be tested for both – no bad thing as gonorrhoea is very often silent in women and serious if untreated.

A fair proportion of cases of trichomonas can be caught, however, by self-contamination alone. It is important to realise this as much grief has been experienced by monogamous couples who, on the diagnosis of trichomonas, presume that one or the other must have been unfaithful. Just like thrush and E. coli, trichomonas can make its way into the vagina because of poor hygiene – wiping from back to front instead of front to back after using the toilet and having anal then vaginal stimulation or sex without washing the relevant extremity first. Less easily avoidable, however, is the possibility of catching trichomonas from upward faecal splashes, if the previous user of the toilet was harbouring the infection. This is, however, a rather rare source of infection.

As trichomonas can survive outside the body for a few hours, if it is somewhere suitably warm and moist, it can be caught by sharing a towel or flannel with someone who has it. It can sometimes be contracted from

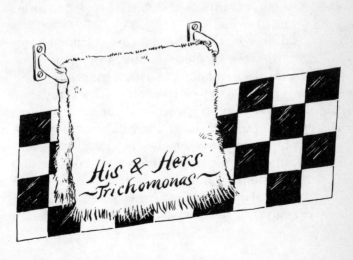

His & Hers ~Trichomonas~

swimming pools, particularly if you stay in your wet swimsuit for a while afterwards, and in rare cases from lavatory seats.

As trichomonas likes a less acidic environment than the normal vagina, it is most likely to be contracted when the acidity is lowered, such as before a period.

WHAT ARE THE RISKS IF UNTREATED?

Infection with trichomonas has been documented as one of the possible risk factors for cervical cancer (see Chapter 7), because it can cause changes in the cells of the cervix similar to those that are known to be pre-cancerous. However, when it is trichomonas alone that is responsible for such cell irregularities, they quickly return to normal once the infection is treated – one excellent reason for seeking early treatment.

Trichomonas harboured during the third term of pregnancy may increase the risk of premature, low birthweight babies, who are generally more susceptible to infections. An American study found that women suffering trichomonas for some time in their sixth to ninth month had a three or four times higher risk of this than women without any infection or with thrush or chlamydia (see Chapter 6) alone.

It is possible, too, that in some cases of pneumonia or respiratory distress in young babies, the agent responsible is trichomonas passed on from a mother during pregnancy. Doctors from the Netherlands recommended in a British medical journal that trichomonas should be tested for whenever a baby's breathing problems have no clearly identifiable cause.

Finally, men don't necessarily get off scot-free of consequences from trichomonas. In rare cases it can cause temporary infertility if present in large quantities in the semen. Fertility is restored as soon as the infection is treated.

WHAT IS THE TREATMENT?

Trichomonas is treated with an antiprotozoan, most usually metronidazole, except in early pregnancy. It may be prescribed in 200mg tablets to be taken three times a day with food for seven days or, less inconveniently, in a single 2g oral dose. Alcohol should be avoided, because it can make you feel ill while taking metronidazole, and so should sex, because of risk of reinfection. Your partner or partners need to take the treatment too – most genito-urinary clinics will prescribe for them without their needing to go for examination.

Some women are very susceptible to trichomonal infection. The good news for them is that there is now a vaccine available to reduce the likelihood of recurrences. In trials at St Mary's Hospital in London, of 100 women who had a history of trichomonal infection and who were given a three injection course of the vaccine, only five had a recurrence in the next eight months, compared with 32 out of 100 given only a placebo.

HOW TO HELP YOURSELF

Obviously you can reduce the risks of sexually transmitted trichomonas by having sex only with one partner, who also only has sex with you. If you do have a rather active sex life with more than one partner, avoid using the IUD as your form of contraception. IUDs increase the likelihood of contracting genital infections generally.

Do all the right hygienic things, like wiping from front to back and avoiding organisms from the anus being passed to the vagina by a penis, finger or vibrator. To be on the safe side, don't sit on public toilet seats or, alternatively, put clean tissue paper down first. Don't share other people's towels or flannels or dive into their wet swimming costumes because you have forgotten your own. Wear loose clothing and cotton underwear, so that air can circulate and keep you cool and dry. Remember, trichomonas likes warm, damp places best.

If you have any suspicious symptoms, it would be wise to seek an early investigation.

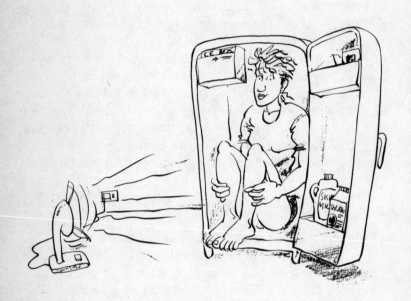

6.
CHLAMYDIA

WHAT IS IT?

Chlamydia (full name *Chlamydia trachomatis*) is the
most common sexually transmitted disease in the
Western world. It has been estimated that there are
probably 170,000 new cases a year and innumerable
women's lives have been ruined on account of it. Yet very
many women have never even heard of it.

This is not so surprising as it seems. Chlamydia is a
bacterium but an odd one. It contains no living cells and,
more like a virus, is dependent on the energy produced
by the cells of its host (i.e. us) for it to grow and reproduce.
It cannot be detected by the usual means for detecting
bacteria and so for many years was not detected at all.
It is only in recent years, with more sophisticated
diagnostic procedures, that chlamydia has been realised
to be so widespread. Chlamydia can live in various parts
of the body, including the liver, the lungs and the throat,
but in adults it is almost always sexually transmitted
and is found mainly in the sexual organs. It is highly
infectious, as there is about a 70 per cent chance of
catching it from a partner who has it. Women who are
diagnosed with gonorrhoea are more than likely to be
harbouring chlamydia too.

WHAT ARE THE SYMPTOMS IN WOMEN?

This is where the big trouble starts. As many as two thirds of the women with chlamydia may have no symptoms at all. When it does produce symptoms, these are likely to be a slight increase in vaginal discharge, caused by the cervix becoming inflamed (cervicitis), soreness and a frequent need to pee with pain when you do. These symptoms, of course, are similar to those caused by a combination of other vaginal or genital infections, such as thrush, herpes and cystitis, so the diagnosis may be missed if women are not fully tested. Chlamydia can also infect the rectum, giving rise to painful bowel movements, occasional bleeding and burning sensations. If transferred to the eye, which it can be by hand, you are likely to suffer a nasty conjunctivitis.

It doesn't end there, unfortunately. If you don't have symptoms, the infection can travel on up in its own good time and wreak havoc with the reproductive organs (see below). It used to be thought that women who had had hysterectomies were not at risk of harbouring chlamydia in the vagina, but this has been proved wrong. But even though they need no longer fear for their fertility, they still need treatment, as they can suffer other symptoms such as inflammation of the vagina and can infect sexual partners who can then pass this dreadful disease on.

WHAT ARE THE SYMPTOMS IN MEN?

It is now known that the insidious chlamydia is responsible for about half the cases of non-specific urethritis (NSU) in men. NSU is the most common sexually transmitted disease for which men seek treatment and, as its name implies, it is caused by unidentifiable organisms. Now with the implication of chlamydia, we do know the cause in the majority of cases. But chlamydial urethritis is symptomless in one in ten men. Much of the rest of NSU may be caused by obscure organisms called mycoplasma, also sexually transmitted and having similar effects on the female, if untreated, to chlamydia.

The usual symptoms of NSU – or NGU (a slightly more specific term standing for non-gonococcal urethritis or 'we don't know what it is but we know it isn't gonorrhoea' in men are a clear, but not particularly profuse, mucus discharge from the penis and a tingling sensation when peeing. These symptoms are usually experienced within two or three weeks of catching the infection, but it is not uncommon for nothing to be noticed till as long as six weeks after sex with an infected person.

HOW DO YOU GET IT?

In adults, chlamydia is almost always acquired via sex with a partner who has it. It can, however, be transferred from the genitals to the eye and, less certainly, vice versa. Once it has been caught, even if it is symptomless for years, there is no chance of it going away again by itself. It can instead stick around to do damage to the fallopian tubes. In this it is unfortunately aided by gynaecological operations, such as having an IUD fitted, an abortion or a D and C (dilatation and curettage), as the infection can then be introduced to the higher reproductive organs.

WHAT ARE THE RISKS IF UNTREATED?

The risks are serious for any woman who wants to have children. Chlamydia causes cervicitis, inflammation of the cervix, and, if untreated, may ascend into the womb lining and the fallopian tubes, causing an infection there – salpingitis. It is now realised that a high proportion of cases of pelvic inflammatory disease (PID) and infertility resulting from blocked fallopian tubes is caused

55

by chlamydia. Because it so often remains symptomless, a number of women may only discover that they have been harbouring chlamydia when they try and fail to get pregnant and start having infertility tests.

PID is the term used to describe a range of pelvic infections, affecting any or all of the womb, the fallopian tubes and the ovaries. Doctors are seeing well over 12,000 new cases a year and, according to Swedish research, a single attack can be sufficient to cause infertility in some. Three quarters of the women who have three attacks are likely to become sterile. So it is very important to act on the early signs, if any, and take sensible preventive measures (see below).

If women have chlamydia when they are pregnant (it has been estimated that between two and 37 per cent of women do have a chlamydia infection during pregnancy), they are at higher risk of an ectopic pregnancy, having a premature or stillborn baby or a baby who dies shortly after birth, as well as having a greater chance of suffering pelvic infection themselves after delivery.

Babies born to mothers with chlamydia have nearly a 50 per cent risk of being infected with the disease themselves, either in the form of an eye infection (chlamydial conjunctivitis) or pneumonia. The conjunctivitis usually develops when the baby is about a week old and if its causes are not identified and the wrong or insufficient antibiotics are given, the cornea of the baby's eye may be permanently scarred and vision affected. Pneumonia, which can be fatal, may not develop for several weeks and as it is only relatively recently that chlamydia has been identified as a possible cause (between 10 and 20 per cent of babies born to mothers with chlamydia are likely to get it), many doctors may misdiagnose the causes and consequently give the wrong treatment.

Chlamydia may also be implicated in some cases of

the early abnormal changes in the cells of the cervix which precede, if unchecked, the development of cervical cancer. Researchers have found chlamydia present in a number of women with pre-cancerous cell changes, although this does not of course pinpoint chlamydia as the cause. It may, however, be one of several risk factors – such as starting sex at an early age, several pregnancies, numerous partners or a partner who has had numerous partners, a history of various sexually transmitted diseases and smoking – all of which can raise one's likelihood of getting cervical cancer. Some researchers have also found, however, that treatment for the chlamydia can reverse any abnormalities in the cells.

It all sounds very alarming and unfortunately it is. Men do not necessarily escape lightly either, although their risk of suffering complications is far lower. Sometimes men who have NSU develop Reiter's disease which can cause conjunctivitis, arthritis (usually in the ankles) and sometimes ulcers on the penis and in the mouth. It appears that some people are pre-disposed to developing Reiter's disease and that chlamydia may be a trigger rather than a cause.

Chlamydia can also cause infertility in men because it can lead to infection in the collecting tube for sperm at the top of the testicle. However, men would only become infertile if both testicles were affected and, for some fortunate but unknown reason, that rarely occurs.

WHAT IS THE TREATMENT?

Ironically, the treatment for chlamydia is simple and effective – once it is given. The greater problem has always been that chlamydia may not be tested for early enough, especially if a woman has no symptoms. Till fairly recently, many clinics had no laboratory facilities available to them for testing for chlamydia. Fortunately, with the development of simpler, quicker tests and professional protest about inadequate concern on the part of government, testing for chlamydia is now much more widely available.

The usual treatment, for both partners, is three 500 mg tablets of oxytetracycline or an equivalent antibiotic daily for seven days and sometimes in addition two 400 mg tablets of metronidazole daily for five days. In pregnancy, erythromycin is given instead of oxytetracycline.

The doctors at genito-urinary clinics are extremely alert to chlamydia nowadays. But many general practitioners and even some gynaecologists may not be aware of its prevalence. They may prescribe ampicillin or metronidazole alone for women with symptoms of PID, but this only suppresses the symptoms and does not get rid of the chlamydia.

HOW TO HELP YOURSELF

If you have any kind of vaginal discharge, soreness, unusually frequent need to pee and pain when you do, always go for a check up.

Preferably go to a genito-urinary clinic where they are far more likely to do a whole range of tests. If you do go to your own doctor and he just presumes you have thrush or cystitis and treats you accordingly, this really isn't good enough. Either insist on being fully tested or, if you do submit and just take the treatment, go back at once if the symptoms still persist afterwards.

Watch out for any early signs of PID. If you have low pelvic pains that persist for a week, go and insist on being investigated. Do *not* settle for being given ampicillin or metronidazole if you have not been checked for chlamydia first and found to be free of it.

Sometimes the low pelvic pains are the only symptoms of PID you will suffer, so don't dismiss them as unimportant. However, there may be some bleeding between periods and bleeding after sex, though remember there can be other reasons for breakthrough bleeding between periods. You are quite likely to have breakthrough bleeding if you are on the progestogen only (POP or mini) pill. But don't ignore it even then, if it is enough to concern you, because you are at higher risk of PID when you use the mini-pill anyway.

Your general practitioner may think, if he is not overly enlightened, that if you have breakthrough bleeding while on the contraceptive pill (any kind), it just doesn't suit you and you need another brand. He may be right and one pill change is reasonable. If it keeps happening, however, ask to be referred to a gynaecologist. Or you can take matters into your own hands by going to a genito-urinary clinic, to which you don't ever need to be referred, telling them your symptoms and asking if you should be tested for chlamydia. You only have to have pelvic pains and most genito-urinary clinics will test you at once!

If there really are no testing facilities for chlamydia in your area and you are obliged to rely on your general practitioner, ask, if you have *any* of the above symptoms, for your treatment to cover the possibility of chlamydia (i.e. the correct drug regime, as stated above).

If you have to have an abortion, it is worth going to a genito-urinary clinic first to ask for a test for chlamydia – and tell them why. In a recent study, 10 per cent of women undergoing abortion were found to be harbouring chlamydia.

Avoid the IUD as your method of contraception. Or, if it really is the only option left to you for whatever reason, be checked for chlamydia before you have the IUD inserted. If it is present, it will quite likely be carried upwards during the surgical procedure to where it can do most damage.

Pill users are at two or three times the normal risk of getting chlamydia. It used to be thought that the pill was protection against PID because it lessens the likelihood of blocked tubes caused by gonococcal infection (gonorrhoea). However, it does not have a protective effect against chlamydial infection, as recently discovered, although many general practitioners may not yet realise this. So if you have ever suffered PID and are prescribed the pill as a preventive measure to reduce your likelihood of getting it again, don't go for it.

Finally, be realistic about your lifestyle. If you have or have had a number of sexual partners, of course you are at higher risk because you have that many more chances of being infected by someone who unknowingly has chlamydia. But it isn't just what you do, it is what your partner does too. Even if you are absolutely monogamous, if your partner is not – even if he perhaps just has the very occasional one night stand when abroad on business – you are inevitably at risk. So make sure you are alert to any odd symptoms, however clean your own lifestyle, and have occasional checks.

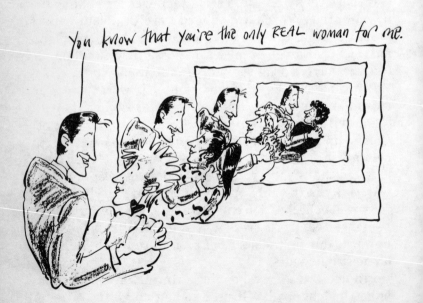

A good preventive measure is to opt for a barrier contraceptive (the diaphragm or condom) used with a spermicide containing the active ingredient Nonoxynol-9. The contraceptive sponge also contains this. Nonoxynol-9 has been found to inhibit the growth of several organisms, including the one that causes chlamydia.

If your partner has any symptoms of NSU, urge him to go for a check and go yourself. If you or he is diagnosed as having chlamydia, it is vital you are both treated. And it is vital that you inform anyone else you could have passed it on to, so that they can be treated, however embarrassing the circumstances may be.

As said earlier, chlamydia is horribly infectious and can cause an enormous amount of grief if not caught early. As so often it doesn't cause any symptoms, we all have to take a fair amount of the responsibility ourselves to thwart it.

7.
GENITAL WARTS

WHAT ARE THEY?

Genital warts are one of the new worries of the '80s. They have been around for a very long time, but it is only recently that they have been linked with an increased incidence of cervical cancer.

Warts are caused by a group of viruses which are described under the umbrella term of human papillomavirus (HPV). The virus changes skin cells that normally form flat skin into cells that form heaped-up skin, resulting in a wart. There are many different types of HPV and each produces warts of a distinct appearance. HPV 1, for instance, causes plantar warts, the type that is found on the soles of the feet. HPV 6, 11, 16 and 18 are the four that are associated with genital warts, also known medically as *condyloma acuminatum*.

Genital warts can be found anywhere around the external genitalia and the anus in both sexes and, in women, also on the walls of the vagina and the cervix. Warts are particularly fond of moisture, which helps them to spread, so they are often to be found in association with a vaginal discharge caused by another infection. They can sometimes be found in the mouth.

In recent years, there has been a huge increase in patients at genito-urinary clinics being diagnosed with warts. In 1984, 45,437 new patients were treated – twice the number of ten years ago. But whereas ten years ago, genital warts were seen as not much more than a nuisance, it now appears that they may be much more nasty than that (see below) and are certainly not to be ignored at any price.

WHAT ARE THE SYMPTOMS IN WOMEN?

The most obvious symptom, of course, is the wart itself or a whole group of them scattered around the genital and anal area. Unfortunately, however, flat (early stage) warts on the cervix cannot be seen by a doctor without the aid of a special microscope called a colposcope which shows in clear detail the cells of the cervix. These colposcopes are most usually available to gynaecologists, but to only a few large genito-urinary clinics. This is unfortunate because most clinics would be only too keen to have a colposcope, but are prevented by lack of NHS funds. At the present time, therefore, flat warts on the cervix may be missed in many cases.

The only other symptom in women is that often, as mentioned earlier, they may have an abnormal vaginal discharge at the same time, not caused by the warts but creating an environment conducive to their continued existence.

Genital warts may become particularly profuse in pregnancy, because during pregnancy the body's immune system is suppressed and women are more susceptible to infection.

WHAT ARE THE SYMPTOMS IN MEN?

Uncircumcised men are more likely to have warts, because warts like to congregate under the foreskin of the penis where it is more moist and warm. But they can be found anywhere on the penis and around the anus (up the anus, too, if the men are homosexual or bisexual) and sometimes they can spread to the tip of the urethra. But they don't produce much in the way of symptoms, except occasional itching. Men too can have flat warts on the penis which can only be detected with a colposcope.

HOW DO YOU GET THEM?

Genital warts are sexually transmitted. If your partner has genital warts, visible or not, you have a 60 per cent chance of getting them as well. Genital warts can also be passed to the mouth by oral sex.

WHAT ARE THE RISKS IF UNTREATED?

In recent years, more and more evidence has come to light that genital warts may be associated with the increased incidence of cervical cancer, particularly in women under 34. New technology has enabled laboratories to detect the presence of the wart virus (from cervical smears) in much cervical pre-cancer and cancer. HPV 16 and 18 seem to be found more usually in cancerous changes that progress to malignancy while HPV 6 and 11 are associated with lower risk and pre-cancerous changes that are more likely to regress on their own.

This does not mean, however, that if you have or have ever had genital warts, you are going to get cervical cancer. It is unlikely that genital warts alone are responsible. They are one risk factor which, in conjunction with others such as starting sex early (when the cervix is immature), a high number of pregnancies, numerous sexual partners or one partner who himself has other partners, a history of other sexually transmitted diseases and smoking, can increase one's chances of having cervical cancer.

The increase in incidence of genital warts has, however, certainly corresponded with the alarming increase in cervical cancer of a particularly aggressive kind in young women. In the last 17 years, there has been a 60 per cent increase in pre-cancerous cervical lesions (early abnormal changes in cervical cells which may regress spontaneously or progress to invasive cancer if untreated). There are 2000 deaths from cervical cancer each year. According to one consultant gynaecologist who is an expert on cervical cancer, the wart virus has been found in over 70 per cent of women with cervical cancer or pre-cancer. Recently a large Australian study found that of 1000 women carrying the wart virus 30 went on to develop cervical cancer, a figure 15 times higher than expected. Young women were particularly at risk, especially if they were under 25 when the wart virus was first diagnosed.

Cervical cancer used to be suffered mainly by older women and it took years for abnormal cell changes to progress and become malignant. Now, alarmingly, it is younger women who are at increased risk, because of the new aggressive form of the disease, perhaps associated with the wart virus, which can progress in months. One laboratory found that while 84 per cent of women who had had positive smears (clear changes in cervical cells) went on as expected to develop cancer quickly, so did nearly half of the women whose smears had shown only mild abnormalities and a third of those who had even milder irregularities. Thus the standard government recommendation that cervical smears should be taken at five year intervals is clearly out of date, although currently it still stands.

The horrible irony is that cervical cancer is one of medicine's success stories. If treated during the pre-invasive stage there is a 95 per cent cure rate. The treatment is so simple that the cancer can be removed in minutes, with no need for major surgery and with no adverse effects on future fertility either. But if left it can be lethal. Sixty per cent of untreated pre-cancerous lesions are likely to go on to become invasive (see below, in the section on treatment).

It is worth mentioning that some genito-urinary specialists and gynaecologists think that the likely link between genital warts and the incidence of cervical cancer has been somewhat over-played. They feel that it could be just the current 'fashion' and that genital warts may no more strongly implicated, in the end, than other sexually transmitted diseases. But, as they *are* the current concern, this chapter is as appropriate as any in which to talk about the treatment for cervical cancer as well as the treatment for warts.

WHAT IS THE TREATMENT?

There are several methods of removing warts. They can be removed by laser (in which a very concentrated beam of light vaporises the virus-infected cells), but this is rather expensive. They can be frozen off with liquid nitrogen (a method called cryosurgery). In very many clinics the first line of approach is to apply some caustic substance to the warts to burn them off or to apply podophylline, an extract from a fungus which has the effect of stopping the cell infected with the virus from dividing and growing. The treatment has to be repeated every few days until the warts go away. Some genital warts can be very persistent and keep coming back – and obviously they are more likely to do so if your partner still has his. Both of you must be treated.

If the wart virus has shown up on a smear (the removal of cells by scraping them from the cervix for examination) or some abnormality (normally termed *dysplasia*) is found in your cervical cells, you should be referred to a gynaecologist for colposcopy. The colposcope, as mentioned before, is a special microscope which is inserted into the vagina so that the doctor can see the exact shape of the cervical cells. It is no more uncomfortable than an internal examination and only takes about ten minutes, with no need for any anaesthetic. Tiny samples of cell tissue may be taken (this is called a punch biopsy) for examination more fully under a microscope.

If the abnormality does warrant treatment, this is now most usually done by laser, by cryosurgery (freezing off with liquid nitrogen), or by diathermy (the use of heat to burn off abnormal cells). Only diathermy requires a general anaesthetic and a few days in hospital. The other methods can be done in out-patient departments, under local anaesthetic.

In cases where the abnormality has already become cancerous but has not gone beyond the outer layers of the cervix (a stage known as *carcinoma in situ*) or in areas of the country where colposcopy is not available, a cone biopsy may be carried out. This is the excision of a larger area of cervical cells and is carried out under general anaesthetic. It should not affect fertility. However, it is certainly not ideal for a cone biopsy to be done as a method of diagnosis, just because of the lack of availability of colposcopes.

If the cancer has spread beyond the outer layers of the cervix into the pelvis, it is termed *invasive* and treatment will have to be more aggressive, perhaps including radiation as well as surgery. It is an unnecessary tragedy for any cervical cancer to be allowed to progress so far and much fault lies with the inadequacy of our cervical screening services. It is estimated that if smears were taken every two or three years, 90 per cent of cervical cancers could be prevented. In Denmark, where all women in the at risk age groups are screened every two to three years, incidence of the cancer has dropped by two thirds. We need to carry on the campaign for better services but, in the meantime, we can also take a number of preventive measures ourselves.

HOW TO HELP YOURSELF

If you have any genital warts that you can see, go and get them treated at a genito-urinary clinic and make sure your partner or partners go too.

If you have had genital warts, remember that they can recur spontaneously and particularly like warmth and dampness. So, if you ever get a vaginal infection, such as thrush, or any other genital infection, it is best to be checked out again for warts as well.

Experts now think that women with a history of certain sexually transmitted diseases should have cervical smears every year, not every five years. If you have had warts or herpes and especially both, do your best to get a yearly smear. Your own doctor will only do it if he or she is sympathetic because general practitioners are only paid for taking smears at five year intervals from women over 35. However, family planning clinics take smears from younger women and so do genito-urinary clinics. If you are not at any higher risk, still make sure of having a regular smear – at least every five years.

Wherever you have your smear taken, you should take responsibility yourself for checking the result. There have been some frightening reports in the press in recent times of women who were not notified of positive results and who therefore did not get treatment in time. Even if your doctor says that you will be notified only if your smear is positive, ask when you can ring for yourself to find out the actual result.

If you are told that your smear shows some mild abnormalities but that you should not worry and should just come for another in six months or a year, ask to be referred to a gynaecologist *now*. The experts say that abnormalities, however mild, should be dealt with at once and not left to see whether they progress or not. However, it is difficult for general practitioners if the area is not one in which they are especially interested, so they may not see the need for instant action. It is true, unfortunately, that not all gynaecologists may see the need for instant action either, especially as it could mean a workload of such large proportions that they couldn't cope. But it is worth a try.

You can, of course, reduce your risk of cervical cancer by being somewhat circumspect about your sex life. Cervical cancer is not a disease caught only by 'promiscuous' women and it is very unfortunate that that image has taken such hold. You can be unlucky enough to get it even if you and your partner are totally monogamous. But you will inevitably be at higher risk if you do have a large number of sexual partners or if your partner does.

If you do have an active sex life with more than one partner, you can help protect yourself by opting for barrier methods of contraception, such as the diaphragm with spermicide or the condom. One heartening American study found that 136 out of 139 women whose smears showed up abnormalities in the cells recovered completely without any treatment once their partners started using the sheath.

If you are a smoker, you can eliminate at least one of the risks at once if you want to enough – by stopping smoking. Smoking can have an adverse effect on the cells of the cervix.

Finally, a preventive measure that doesn't hurt. Eat more fruit and vegetables containing beta-carotene, which is used by the body, when needed, to form vitamin A. Several studies have shown that beta-carotene in the diet can help protect against certain cancers, including cancer of the lung and cancer of the cervix. Vegetables rich in beta-carotene include carrots (very high), broccoli, green leafy vegetables, sweet potatoes and tomatoes. Apricots are the best source in fruit but peaches and prunes are good value too. Do *not* think you will be doing the sensible thing by taking a vitamin A supplement.

Vitamin A can be toxic in large quantities whereas beta-carotene does nothing more than turn you slightly orange if you happen to eat too much and that would take a lot!

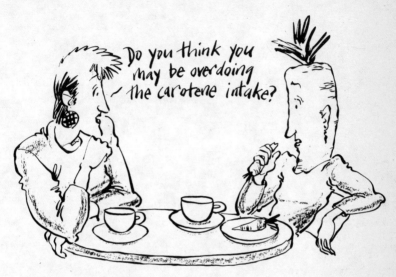

8.
HERPES

WHAT IS IT?

Herpes it an extremely common virus. There are four
different types but only two need concern us here, as only
these two, HSV (herpes simplex virus) 1 and 2 can give
rise to genital herpes. HSV 1 is more familiar to us as
cold sores, which usually appear on the lips and
occasionally on the nose or cheeks. Somewhere between
70 and 90 per cent of the population have been infected
by the cold sore virus at some time, usually in childhood.
Once we have been infected we remain carriers of the
virus for life because it doesn't go away – it travels up
into a nerve where it usually stays dormant. However,
it can, when it wants to, travel down again and cause a
recurrence of cold sores if we haven't built up enough
resistance against it. Probably one fifth of the population
suffer frequent recurrences. It used to be thought that
HPV 1 and HPV 2, which causes genital herpes, were
rather more distinct from each other than they actually
are. But it now seems that up to 60 per cent of cases of
genital herpes are in fact caused by HPV 1, transferred
to the genitals via oral sex.

Genital herpes appear most usually on the penis and
around the anus in men and on and around the vaginal
lips, the clitoris, inside the vagina, on the cervix and

around the anus in women. But they can often also be found on the thighs and buttocks. There were 20,000 new cases reported in 1984, double that of five years ago but probably in large part because more people are now aware of what it is and seek a diagnosis. There are in fact likely to be as many as a million sufferers at any one time, because a great many cases are still not reported or not even noticed. Genital herpes caused quite a scare a few years ago, because it suddenly seemed present in 'epidemic' proportions in America and sharply on the increase here. The alarm was fuelled by the fact that herpes is incurable. However, it is only an unfortunate minority of people who suffer very recurrent attacks and, as much can be done by sufferers themselves to reduce the likelihood of attacks and manage the possible risks (e.g. during childbirth – see below), it may in fact have less serious consequences than many other genital infections. It is, however, extremely unpleasant and, for those who do have recurrent attacks, it can have serious effects on social and sexual relationships.

WHAT ARE THE SYMPTOMS IN WOMEN?

Genital herpes usually shows up as clusters of little red spots with white blisters somewhere in the genital region. However it is quite possible for it to appear as a tiny single spot. Herpes takes some little while to show after contact with a person who has it – usually between two and 20 days, with an average incubation period of six.

The little blisters burst and form painful open sores. At this stage it can be excruciatingly painful to pee, as the acidic urine comes into contact with them and creates a burning sensation – often mistaken in the first instance for cystitis. Sometimes the sores themselves become infected by bacteria and there can be painful swelling in the lymph glands in the groin. Women may often find that they have an abnormal vaginal discharge.

The first attack of genital herpes is almost always the worst, as it can be accompanied in some people by a high fever. And yet others have no symptoms that they notice at all, not even the blisters because they may be hidden in the folds of the vaginal lips. The time from the appearance of the blisters to when they burst, crust over and then heal is usually 16 to 18 days for a first attack and about eight days for any subsequent ones.

Recurrent attacks are much milder because the body has had a chance to build up some resistance. For about 30 per cent of people the first attack is the last. Others may range from a few attacks in a lifetime to a couple of attacks a year to, for a minority, an attack almost every month. Experts now believe that people who have low recurrences are more likely to have been infected by HPV 1, via someone's cold sores, rather than by the genital herpes strain itself, HPV 2. In recurrences, there is no fever and usually there are fever lesions on the genitals.

For most people an attack of herpes is heralded a day or two before by some warning sign, known as the prodome. These signs vary from individual to individual and may include an itch, a tingling sensation, a dull ache in the groin, tenderness, a feeling of pain in the pelvis and/or legs or just a sensation that something is about to happen. Such signs are not likely to mean anything to you the first time around, but if you have had an attack of herpes once, they are very useful warnings of another. Inevitably, however, once you have been diagnosed as having had herpes, you will be aware of all sorts of odd sensations in the genital region, because you have heightened awareness of what may be happening down there. Most of these, fortunately, will not be anything to do with herpes, just false alarms which subside once you start to relax and not worry so much that you are about to have a new attack every day.

WHAT ARE THE SYMPTOMS IN MEN?

Symptoms are the same in men. Whereas some women may experience an abnormal vaginal discharge, men may notice a mucous discharge from the penis, if the urethra has been infected, as well as sores.

HOW DO YOU GET IT?

Genital herpes is most commonly acquired through sex with a person who has herpes during its active stage. The virus is shed just before the blisters erupt and while the sores are present. Some people, however, do have asymptomatic herpes, which means they do not get blisters but they still shed the virus. It passes on to a partner by entering through any breaks in the skin or through particularly soft parts called mucous membranes, which line bits of the body such as the genitals and the eyes. Although it is indeed infectious, it is actually by no means as easily transmitted as some other genital infections. According to one estimate, you have a 15 per cent chance of catching herpes if you have sex with someone who is shedding the herpes virus at that time. As mentioned above, you can also get genital herpes from someone's cold sores, if you have oral sex with them.

Herpes can live outside the body for a little while, so it is indeed possible to catch it from towels and, according to some evidence, from toilet seats. You can give it to yourself, of course, if you touch a cold sore on your face and then touch your genitals.

When you have had genital herpes once, there are a number of trigger factors which may precipitate a subsequent attack. Again, these vary from individual to individual but they include being over-stressed and run down, having a fever or another infection and the genitals being exposed to sunlight (e.g. during nude sunbathing). Some women say that when they are having a period they are most vulnerable to an attack, while for others the act of sex can do it because of the bruising and friction. Fortunately, however, there are steps we can take to reduce the likelihood of a recurrence in most of these cases.

WHAT ARE THE RISKS IF UNTREATED?

Herpes cannot be treated in the sense of cured but the risks to health arising from herpes can be minimised by good management (see below).

There is evidence that herpes on the cervix is a risk factor for cervical cancer. That means not that herpes can cause cervical cancer but that its presence, along with several other risk factors, may increase your likelihood of getting it (see Chapter 7).

Because herpes can be transmitted by the finger, there is a high risk of transferring it to the eye, causing conjunctivitis and ulceration that can lead, if not checked by anti-viral drugs, to impaired or loss of corneal vision and permanent scarring. Herpes simplex virus is the main cause of corneal blindness in the Western world. Infection of the eye is far more likely to occur through touching a cold sore on the lip and then the eye, but it can also be the result of the transfer of infection from the genitals – particularly likely during lovemaking. In the same way that cold sores and genital herpes can recur, so can herpetic eye infections, with stress, illness, menstruation and ultraviolet light again being possible trigger factors.

Women with herpes are at particular risk when they are pregnant, with an increased likelihood of miscarriage and premature birth. They can, unfortunately, pass herpes on to their newborn babies if they have an attack at the time of giving birth, especially if it is a first attack. Even women who have not had a recurrence of herpes for over a year are quite likely to suffer one during pregnancy, particularly in the last three months.

A baby born with herpes usually has lesions all over its body and the disease is fatal in 60 per cent of cases. Those that survive are likely to have permanent brain and/or eye damage. This terrible risk is to be avoided at all costs and in most cases it can be (see section on treatment).

WHAT IS THE TREATMENT?

As already mentioned, there is no cure as yet for herpes. If you have symptoms which you think may be herpes, you should go as soon as possible to a genito-urinary clinic for diagnosis. The virus is usually shed when the blisters have just broken and later than that it may not be possible to make a diagnosis either way.

There are a few anti-viral drugs which seem to relieve many of the symptoms of the herpes attack and speed healing. Unfortunately, none can claim to prevent recurrences although they may reduce them. One of the drugs most commonly used is acyclovir (Zovirax) which comes in tablet form and also as a cream. If the cream is applied as soon as any itching or tingling starts, blisters do not develop at all in a third of cases. As virus shedding is reduced when the cream is used, there is also less chance of spreading the disease elsewhere on yourself or to someone else. Trials have shown that oral acyclovir given daily as a preventive measure can significantly reduce the likelihood of recurrences, but as this is an expensive measure and may have side effects in the long-term, it is only likely to be advised, if at all, for people who are severely incapacitated by very frequent herpes attacks.

Also commonly used to treat symptoms is inosine pranobex (Imunovir), which seems to work by enhancing the body's own immune system so that it can fight off an attack more quickly. It appears to reduce the number of recurrences.

Various drugs are under trial in the search to find a cure for herpes. There are still hopes for a vaccine and also, now, for an anti-herpes drug based on a synthetic enzyme that can prevent the virus from reproducing. But research is in the very early stages.

Pregnant women who have had herpes are usually seen regularly from 32 weeks up till delivery, for swabs to be taken for HSV culture. If they have an attack close to the time of expected delivery, they can safely be delivered by Caesarian section, as the baby would only come in contact with the herpes virus in the birth canal. Many women choose to have a Caesarian anyway, feeling happier to be on the safe side, but it is perfectly feasible to have a vaginal delivery if there are no herpes lesions present at the time.

HOW TO HELP YOURSELF

As with everything, the more sexual partners you have, the higher your chance of getting herpes. It is worth remembering, however, that genital herpes has as much to do with past lifestyles as with the present one. Even if you are in a totally monogamous relationship now, you or your partner may have been exposed to herpes years previously without ever knowing it and therefore a recurrence for one of you could occur. If that happens, it is not advisable for the injured party to fly off the handle with accusations of unfaithfulness, because they may not be justified at all.

A good protective measure is to use for your contraceptive method the diaphragm or the condom in conjunction with a spermicide that contains Nonoxynol-9. The contraceptive sponge contains this spermicide too. Nonoxynol-9 has been shown to be able to inactivate the herpes virus and thus may reduce your risk. Do not have oral sex with anyone who has cold sores.

If you do get genital herpes, there are precautions you should take to reduce any possible health risks and to minimise recurrences. Experts advise, to be on the safe side, getting a yearly cervical smear. You can go to a genito-urinary clinic, a family planning clinic or your own doctor who, depending on how sympathetic he or she is, may be prepared to take one regularly if you explain the reason.

If you get pregnant, make sure you inform your general practitioner and your obstetrician at the outset that you have had herpes, so that they can keep a special check on you for recurrences later in pregnancy.

If you ever get any inflammation of the eye (conjunctivitis) for which you seek treatment from your doctor, tell him if you have had herpes (genital or cold sores). He may not think to ask and may presume you have an allergy to something and treat you with steroid drops. Perhaps you do have an allergy to something, but if in fact you have a herpes infection of the eye, irreparable damage may be done by treatment with steroids alone. Ask to be seen by an ophthalmologist who will make a proper diagnosis and, if you have a herpetic eye infection, will give you the correct anti-viral drugs.

To help prevent recurrences, make sure that when you have sex, you are well lubricated to avoid abrasion. Use a vaginal lubricant available from chemists, if necessary. Never allow the skin around the genitals to become too dry and sore or too hot and humid. Herpes likes moisture. It helps it spread. Avoid irritating chemicals, such as perfumed soaps and bubble baths, and wear loose cotton underpants.

When you are sunbathing, never do so nude, even if the opportunity allows. Ultra-violet light can be a trigger for some people, so at least keep your bikini bottoms on.

Make sure you have a good diet, with plenty of fresh fruit and vegetables. Various vitamins have an important

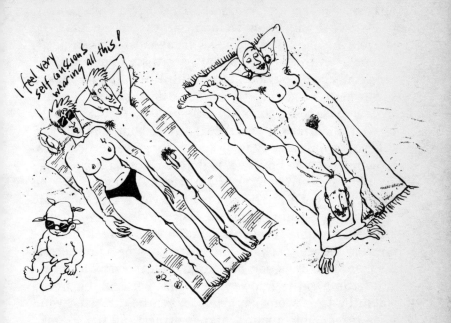

part to play in bolstering our body's natural defences and it is when your defences are down that herpes is most likely to break out.

Try not to get over stressed and learn how to relax if you don't know how. Stress takes its toll on the immune system and leaves you more vulnerable to infections of any kind. But it is important to remember that there is stress and stress. You may like being under pressure and achieve most when the adrenalin is pumping. That is okay, if you end up feeling good. But if you feel over burdened, defeated and anxious about the stress you have to deal with in your life, that is when you are putting yourself at risk. Research shows that it isn't stress itself but stress that is accompanied by depression, which most often precedes a herpes attack.

One important thing not to get stressed about is herpes itself, hard though that may be at first. If you find yourself dwelling on the possibility of having a recurrence and anxiously inspecting yourself for signs, you are more likely to get one. Some women find they often have attacks during periods. However, as most women don't and as even those who do don't get them every period, there may be an element of self-fulfilling prophecy there. If you *expect* to get one then, you will be anxious and this will increase the probability of an attack. You can usually break the pattern if you try to relax about it.

If you are unlucky enough to experience recurrences, remember not to have sex right from the first tingling warning signs (if you get them) right through until the sores are completely healed over. If you are responsible about herpes, you need never risk passing it on. If you are not in a long-term relationship, do not feel that you must announce you have had herpes to a new prospective partner as soon as you meet him. Get to know him first and let him get to know you, so that you can tell him when the time seems right and when he can trust you to be responsible about a herpes attack and not to put him at risk. People who react badly to the news that someone has herpes do so through uninformed fear. If you sound confident about it yourself, you are far more likely to be able to dispel others' worries.

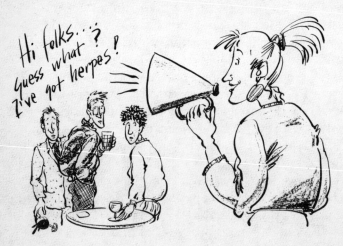

The herpes lesions will heal in their own time and you may only need to go to the doctor for anti-viral tablets or creams if you suffer particularly badly and often. Otherwise you can help yourself by bathing around the vagina in salt water to soothe the soreness and by then keeping the area as dry as possible. It can be less painful to pee if you do so in the shower or run warm water into the bath.

It can help to talk to someone who knows what it is like to have herpes. The Herpes Association is made up of people who do. Their address is 41 North Road, London N7 9DP and you can call their office for information on 01-607 9661 or their helpline for personal advice on 01-609 9061.

9.
LICE AND SCABIES

WHAT ARE THEY?

The pubic or 'crab' louse, the body louse and the head louse are all members of the same family of sucking lice. As its name would imply, the pubic louse is found mainly in the pubic region and around the anus. Its hind legs have claws which hang on to the pubic hairs and which render it faintly crablike in appearance, thus its nickname. There are usually more females than males present, which is unfortunate as the females lay a prodigious number of eggs. They are very small, but possible to see with the naked eye.

Scabies is caused by mites. Mites are smaller than lice and have eight legs, some of them ending in things that look like suckers. Unlike lice, they like to lay their eggs under the skin, so they dig themselves a hole in the outer layer. The genital area is only one of a number of areas of the body which the mite finds attractive.

WHAT ARE THE SYMPTOMS?

The symptoms for both are the same in men and women. With lice, you are likely to have an itch which comes on mainly at night, but some people don't even get that. The itch can be mild or extremely irritating and sometimes there is a rash or tiny spots. However, by the time any of these symptoms make themselves apparent, the lice are likely to have been settled in for a month. In fact, the symptoms are thought to be not symptoms as such but an allergic reaction to their established presence. Of course, the other sign of lice is a glimpse of a louse itself but this is rare.

You are even less likely to see the mite, but it induces similar allergic symptoms, again about a month after its arrival. In this case, however, the itching may occur day and night (though worse at night) and can be absolutely maddening, with buttocks, thighs and armpits particularly affected. If the itch gets scratched, as is all too likely, the holes dug by the mites to lay their eggs can become infected by bacteria and cause a rash. Neither lice nor mites jump.

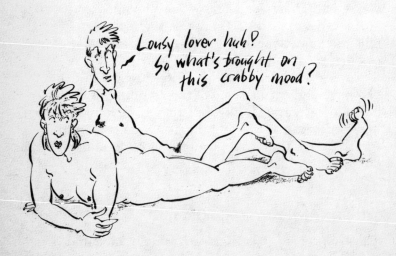

HOW DO YOU GET THEM?

Lice are most commonly transmitted sexually, but it is also possible to get infected if you simply share a bed with someone who has got them. However, the possibility of getting lice from sleeping in a bed previously slept in by someone with lice is extremely remote, unless you are using the bed in shifts, because pubic lice, unlike body lice, cannot survive on their own for more than 24 hours. The likelihood of catching scabies in this way is extremely low too. However, to catch scabies, you certainly don't need to have sex. Close contact is quite sufficient and sharing a bed is the likeliest occasion for transfer.

WHAT ARE THE RISKS IF UNTREATED?

Unpleasant as these infestations are, they do not lead on to anything worse.

WHAT IS THE TREATMENT?

There are special lotions, benzene derivatives, which kill off both and one application is usually enough. For lice, the lotion is applied to the pubic region and for scabies it is applied over the whole body from the neck downwards. Special shampoos used to be used, but these are not ideal as they are washed off too quickly to be fully effective. Partners need to be treated too, but there is no need in either case to do anything special to either clothing or bedding.

HOW TO HELP YOURSELF

Be circumspect about sharing your bed, however platonic your friendship or intent!

10.
GONORRHOEA

WHAT IS IT?

Gonorrhoea is caused by a bacterium known as the gonococcus or *Neisseria gonorrhoeae*, which looks like a coffee bean – in shape not size. It is only possible to see it under a microscope. In women it is the cervix which is almost always infected, but sometimes the urethra, the rectum and less commonly the throat are too. In men it is usually found in the urethra and sometimes also in the throat. In homosexual but rarely heterosexual men, it is also usual to find it in the rectum. Gonorrhoea is highly catching. After one act of sex with a person who has it, there is up to a 90 per cent chance of getting it yourself. Where it hails from originally no one knows, but there are no signs of it wishing to move on. It is the most common sexually transmitted disease in the world.

WHAT ARE THE SYMPTOMS IN WOMEN?

Tragically, there can very often be virtually none. About 50 per cent of women have no symptoms at all and most of the rest will only experience a slight increase in vaginal discharge of no very distinct character. A few women with gonorrhoea have the additional symptom of a certain amount of pain when peeing. Only rarely when the rectum is infected is there any tell-tale discharge from there.

Definite symptoms can manifest themselves much later, but only as a result of the awful complications which occur if the disease is not treated early enough (see below). So, often it is the partner's symptoms which must first alert a woman to the possibility of infection. This is all very well if the partner is a regular one and likely to tell you. One-nighters are not the best source of such information, another very sound reason for keeping down casual contacts. You can also infect someone else with gonorrhoea from the moment you have got it yourself.

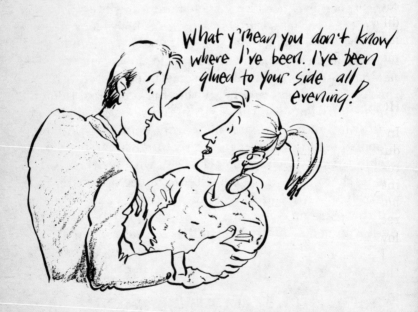

About one third of the women who have gonorrhoea also have gardnerella (see Chapter 3) and nearly half have trichomonas (see Chapter 5), so it may be the symptoms of these which send them to the doctor. And that is a good reason to go to a genito-urinary clinic for diagnosis of any abnormal discharge, if you have any likelihood of having caught a sexually transmitted disease, as they automatically test for gonorrhoea.

WHAT ARE THE SYMPTOMS IN MEN?

It can take up to ten days for men to develop symptoms. These are a thick, yellowish discharge from the penis and an intense pain when peeing. The urethra itself becomes inflamed causing a general sensation of discomfort. Unfortunately, however, it is not unknown for men to have no symptoms either or to have symptoms considerably less severe, as there are now a number of different strains of the gonococcus, which alters itself as necessary to survive in the face of onslaughts from modern medicine.

HOW DO YOU GET IT?

In sexually active adults it is almost always transmitted during sex with a partner who has it. Oral sex is responsible for its being found in the throat. Anal intercourse is the cause of its presence in the rectum in homosexual men, but in a woman involvement of the rectum is far more usually due to the geography of her lower regions.

It is theoretically possible to catch gonorrhoea from the dreaded toilet seat, but for anatomical reasons this is much more of a likelihood (and still a low one) for men than for women. It is, however, perfectly possible for young girls who have never had sex to catch it from an infected towel or something similar. This is because, before puberty, the make-up of the vaginal moisture is different and the gonococcus can then survive (and cause soreness) around the vaginal opening.

WHAT ARE THE RISKS IF UNTREATED?

If untreated in women, gonorrhoea can block the fallopian tubes and lead to infertility or to ectopic pregnancy, because a fertilised egg cannot reach the womb. When the fallopian tubes have been affected, this may be the time when a woman first has symptoms. These may take the form of low pelvic pain and periods may get heavier and more painful. Sometimes a woman gets backache or feels feverish. In rare cases she may suffer peritonitis, an inflammation of the abdomen and pelvis which is potentially lethal if untreated.

Women who have gonorrhoea of the cervix at the time they give birth can infect their baby's eyes with it. Symptoms develop within two days of birth when the eye becomes red and swollen and produces a discharge. If it is not treated, scarring and permanent impairment of vision can result.

Gonorrhoea that is untreated can also give rise to arthritis, as it can affect the joints. In fact, if not recognised for an extremely long time, it can affect virtually every organ in the body, but this is very rare indeed. In men, severe complications are rare because they are more likely to seek treatment early, when they get symptoms.

WHAT IS THE TREATMENT?

Gonorrhoea is somewhat more difficult to diagnose in women, but presents no real problem for the specialist practitioner – again, a good reason for going to a genito-urinary clinic.

Treatment for both partners is with a single dose of oral penicillin, though more may be needed if complications have set in. It is safe to take in pregnancy, but there is an alternative drug for those allergic to penicillin. It is sadly the case that the gonococcus has the ability to develop strains which are resistant to the penicillins commonly used in treatment. This could be catastrophic, except for the fact that the pharmaceutical industry is just about keeping ahead of it with the development of different types of penicillin drugs.

HOW YOU CAN HELP YOURSELF

The fewer sexual partners you have, the less the likelihood of picking up gonorrhoea. If you do have sex regularly or occasionally with men you don't know well – and may not see again – it is desirable to go for check-ups at a genito-urinary clinic at suitable intervals. Do not think that the type of person you have sex with has any bearing on whether you might catch gonorrhoea or not. Men with nice manners or expensive clothes are just as likely to get it as anyone else, if they have an active sex life. But bisexual men are at greater risk, because the incidence of gonorrhoea is high among homosexuals. Go at once for investigation if your partner has any symptoms or if you do yourself.

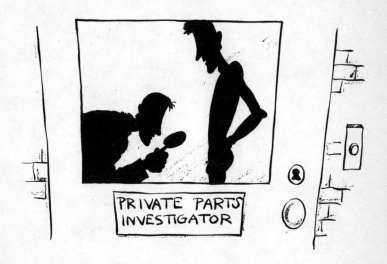

PRIVATE PARTS INVESTIGATOR

Choose your contraception carefully if your lifestyle
puts you at any risk of getting gonorrhoea. The pill can
be protective against gonorrhoea, but its use is associated
with a higher risk of chlamydia (see Chapter 6) which
is just as undesirable. The IUD should not be used, as
it is associated with an increase in genital infections.
Particularly bad are the ones without smooth threads,
as bacteria can use them for a leg up to the higher
reproductive organs. The goodies are the diaphragm or
the condom used with a spermicide containing
Nonoxynol-9, the active ingredient which appears to
inhibit several undesirable organisms, including the
gonococcus. The contraceptive sponge contains
Nonoxynol-9 too.

11.
SYPHILIS

WHAT IS IT?

As far as sexually transmitted diseases go, syphilis has traditionally been thought of as the 'big one'. In fact, it is really rather rare in women nowadays and the men who get it are mainly homosexuals, for reasons explained below. Syphilis is caused by a bacterium called *Treponema pallidum* and known as the treponeme. It is a strangely supple spiral-shaped thing which moves in a rather gymnastic sort of way, according to those who have the benefit of viewing it down a microscope.

The areas of primary infection in women are the lips of the vagina, the clitoris and around the opening to the urethra. Sometimes it can affect the cervix. In men symptoms usually appear on the penis. In both sexes, infection can also occur around the anus, occasionally the mouth and, surprisingly but rarely, the nipples.

It is possible to be born with syphilis if the disease has not been treated in the mother, but that is rare nowadays.

WHAT ARE THE SYMPTOMS IN WOMEN?

It can take as long as three months after sexual contact with an infected person for the symptoms of primary syphilis to show, but more usually something happens within a month. Because the infection, once in the body, blocks the blood supply to the skin in the area where the bacteria entered, the first sign of its presence is a single ulcer or chancre at that spot. The area may be inflamed and the local lymph glands swollen. The ulcer, which is hard underneath to the touch, may be so tiny as to be almost invisible or else stretch to about one centimetre. It is usually painless.

This is all that happens during the next six to eight weeks. In fact, in the majority of cases, the chancre has disappeared by the time that symptoms of secondary syphilis become apparent. Usually a red spotty rash or other sores then appear on various parts of the body. These may disappear quite quickly or stay around for weeks. There may be flat warty-looking growths on the vagina (these are not of the same family as genital warts). Often people get white spots on the tongue. Accompanying all this, there will be fever, aching muscles, bones and joints, a feeling of fatigue and loss of appetite and sometimes even loss of hair, because syphilis attacks the whole body. At this stage it is very common for all the lymph glands and the liver to be enlarged.

Dire as they sound, these symptoms eventually resolve themselves if no treatment is sought or given and the infection becomes latent. In some people it may remain latent until the end of their lives, giving rise to no more symptoms. But in others the disease progresses (see below).

WHAT ARE THE SYMPTOMS IN MEN?

The symptoms are the same in men, except that the first chancre usually appears on the penis, generally on the head of it or the foreskin.

HOW DO YOU GET IT?

Syphilis is acquired sexually. However, it has to enter the skin through a cut or graze which is why homosexual or bisexual men who have anal intercourse, in which tearing of the tissues is much more common, are at higher risk. Ninety per cent of new cases of syphilis are reported by homosexuals. From the time of the appearance of the chancre till about two or three years later, the disease can be passed on sexually, particularly during the time when symptoms are apparent.

WHAT ARE THE RISKS IF UNTREATED?

Tertiary syphilis is nowadays very rare indeed, as the disease is generally caught and treated in its earlier stages. It can affect the skin, the bones, the nervous system (including the brain) leading to dementia and the cardio-vascular system leading to heart failure.

A woman who has syphilis when pregnant can pass on the disease to her baby. If the disease is in its early very infectious stages, she is more likely to miscarry. But if it is in its early latent stage – up to two or three years since she first had symptoms – there is an 80 per cent chance of the baby being born with various defects of the skin, the bones, the eyes and the nervous system. However, congenital syphilis is very rare indeed, because a pregnant woman's blood is tested for syphilis when she first attends the antenatal clinic.

WHAT IS THE TREATMENT?

Syphilis is clearly detected in blood tests and cured quite easily with a course of penicillin injections for 14 days. Penicillin is safe in pregnancy and always effective because the treponeme, which causes syphilis, has not become in any way resistant to it, unlike the gonococcus which causes gonorrhoea. However, there are other drugs available too, for those allergic to penicillin. It is very important that all contacts are treated.

HOW TO HELP YOURSELF

There is little specially that can be done except the usual – avoid frequent changes of sexual partner, although, if you do have several partners, you are much more likely to catch something else rather than syphilis. Bisexual men may present an especial risk however and not only of syphilis, so if you have a partner who is actively bisexual, it is wise to attend a genito-urinary clinic for regular check-ups.

Condoms are protective but not totally. A woman who has syphilis may still infect a man at the base of his penis, the part which isn't covered by the condom, and he then can pass it to you.

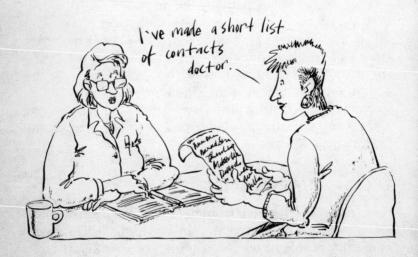

12.
AIDS

WHAT IS IT?

AIDS stands for Acquired Immune Deficiency Syndrome.
It is a breakdown of the body's own immune system,
caused by a virus, and leaves the sufferer, who can be
male or female, vulnerable to rare cancers and
opportunistic infections which do not affect normal
healthy people. It is now also known that the AIDS virus
can attack the brain cells without there ever being any
symptoms of immune-deficiency. To date, AIDS is always
eventually fatal. It was virtually unheard of till 1981
when it suddenly became rife in America, particularly
among homosexuals and intravenous drug users, and was
realised to be widespread in Central Africa and Haiti.
It is speculated that the virus originated in Zaire, spread
to Haiti via a number of the many Haitians who have
recently lived in Zaire and then to America via
homosexuals for whom Haiti has been a popular place
for holidays. It has since spread to Europe and has been
found to be prevalent in other parts of Africa too.

It was not until 1983, however, that the virus which
appears to cause AIDS was identified by two separate
groups of researchers in France and America and given
a name by each of them. The French call it
lymphadenopathy associated virus (LAV), the Americans

human T-cell leukaemia virus (HTLV III). It is now more likely to be known by an international name of HIV (*human immunodeficiency virus*).

Antibodies to the HIV virus can be identified in blood, by means of a blood test. But this merely shows that someone who comes up positive on this test has previously been exposed to the virus and does not prove that they will go on to develop AIDS itself.

It is quite possible for someone to carry the virus for many years without any symptoms at all but during that time he or she can infect other people with it. It is thought that within five years up to 30 per cent of people infected with the virus will develop AIDS symptoms, but as many as 70 per cent may eventually succumb.

At the beginning of 1987, tests became available which can detect the presence of the virus itself and which may perhaps indicate who is at most risk of developing AIDS. Such tests may not be widely available as their usefulness is still under trial, and they need to be used in conjunction with the antibody test, as it is possible to be positive for one and negative for the other.

Because there is as yet no cure for AIDS, many thousands of lives have already been claimed across the world. Experts are desperate to stem the flow by public education on prevention.

WHAT ARE THE SYMPTOMS?

There is no difference in symptoms between men and women and initially they are equally indeterminate in both.

The HIV virus can itself cause symptoms which may later clear up and which do not normally lead on to AIDS. These fairly minor symptoms, known as persistent generalized lymphadenopathy (PGL), are swelling of the lymph glands in the neck and armpits, which last for at least three months.

Others who are infected with the HIV virus may develop what is called AIDS related complex (ARC). The symptoms of this include feeling very overtired and feverish, sudden loss of weight, severe night sweats and persistent diarrhoea. The lymph nodes are enlarged and the person may also start to suffer from extremely severe forms of herpes, oral thrush and shingles – all symptoms associated with mild immuno-deficiency. But nothing fuller may develop.

Symptoms associated with full AIDS itself include all the above but in a much more pronounced and persistent form. The diagnosis of AIDS, however, always depends on the presence of at least one of a number of specific diseases which can arise when the HIV virus is present and the immune system is breaking down. One of the most common is a form of pneumonia caused by an organism which does no harm at all to healthy individuals with immune systems in proper working order. The symptoms are worsening difficulty in breathing and a cough that won't clear.

Another disease very often indicative of AIDS in people positive for the virus is Kaposi's sarcoma, a rare skin cancer which usually shows itself in the development of purplish blotches or bruises anywhere on the skin. Extreme forms of viruses, such as cytomegalovirus, fungi, such as thrush and various bacteria may cause severe intestinal disease, with symptoms from persistent diarrhoea to extreme difficulty swallowing. The virus can also attack the brain, affecting both mood and mental function.

Very many of these symptoms are familiar to us in mild forms and it is all too easy to panic when really there is no cause. In most cases they will indicate some other simpler infection or, sometimes, simply be induced by anxiety about AIDS itself.

HOW DO YOU GET IT?

The virus is only definitely known to be transmitted via semen, vaginal and cervical secretions and blood. It is much less easy to catch than hepatitis B to which it is closest in mode of transmission.

People who were first identified as at high risk were homosexuals, intravenous drug users, haemophiliacs and Haitians. However, it is only likely to be those Haitians whose lifestyles put them at risk who are in any more danger of getting the disease than anyone else. Haemophiliacs were at risk because of blood products which had been infected by donors with AIDS, but this is no longer a risk as blood products are now adequately heat-treated to kill any virus. Still at high risk, however, are homosexuals who practise anal intercourse (easy tearing of the tissues and bleeding during anal sex means that the AIDS virus from an infected partner has easy access into the body) and intravenous drug users who share contaminated hypodermic needles.

Also at risk are people who receive blood transfusions containing infected blood, but this is far less likely to happen now that blood donors are screened for the presence of antibodies to the virus.

Sexual partners of any people who have the HIV virus are at risk of getting it themselves, unless they take preventive steps (see 'How to help yourself'). Women can certainly catch it from infected semen during vaginal intercourse and it is now known that heterosexual men and women can pass the virus to each other this way as easily as gay men may pass it to each other by anal intercourse. In certain parts of Africa, there is an equal split in incidence between the sexes and experts are quite convinced that AIDS will spread through our heterosexual population too, if unchecked. Pregnant women who are infected can easily pass it on to their babies.

You do not catch AIDS from just living in a household where there is a person who suffers from it. The virus is not transferred by casual contact, such as touching or even kissing, according to most experts. Only very little virus has been isolated in saliva and probably is not infectious at all.

More surprisingly, perhaps, it isn't even that easy to get it from cuts or needle pricks that introduce contaminated blood (it is the rare member of a hospital staff who develops symptoms that way – they just receive the full glare of publicity when they do). And there is no evidence that biting or blood-sucking insects can play a part in possible transmissions. The far more infectious hepatitis B is not even transmitted this way.

WHAT ARE THE RISKS IF UNTREATED?

AIDS itself cannot yet be cured. That is, the immune system cannot be returned to full working order. But there are treatments that can be given for all of the aforementioned diseases, such as lung, skin and intestinal diseases, which occur during AIDS. Success is variable. On average, survival after succumbing to pneumonia or the other infections is about nine months and for Kaposi's sarcoma two years. But many may live for as long as, or longer than, four years, after treatment. If the virus attacks the brain, however, it may cause depression that eventually progresses to dementia.

A pregnant woman is at risk, even if she only carries the virus but has no symptoms. Pregnancy itself suppresses the body's immune system (so that the foetus will not be rejected as a foreign body) and may increase the likelihood of the disease becoming active. Two thirds of pregnant women with the virus are likely to have babies with AIDS or the AIDS virus. Some of the risk may be reduced by undergoing Cesarian section rather than vaginal delivery.

WHAT TREATMENTS ARE BEING EXPLORED?

A great deal of research is going on to find an antiviral drug that may reactivate some immune system response and stop the virus replicating, thus preventing disease progression. One current hopeful is the drug azidodeoxythymidine (AZT). Still under trial is the immune system enhancer, inosine pranobex (trade name Imunovir in this country and more commonly used to alleviate symptoms of herpes). However, an antiviral drug may have no effect on AIDS virus in the brain. A number of scientists are working on vaccines to stop AIDS developing but making vaccines against viruses, especially variable ones, is notoriously fraught with difficulties. Even anything that does look hopeful will take years to test because of AIDS' long incubation period.

HOW TO HELP YOURSELF

The best avoidance tactic, obviously, is to avoid casual sex, especially with high risk individuals such as bisexuals and intravenous drug users. However, as the virus is already starting to spread into the general population, it makes sense to use a condom during any casual sexual encounter and, if you are able to, to be sure that your regular partner is faithful to you.

The condom is 85 to 98 per cent safe as a contraceptive, especially if used with a spermicide – preferably one containing Nonoxynol-9, as this has been demonstrated to inactivate even the AIDS virus. However, even if you use some other form of contraception, the condom should be used as well, during casual sex, as a preventive against infection. The biggest risk during vaginal intercourse is that the infection will enter the blood and this is most likely to occur when semen comes in contact with the walls of the vagina, as the skin suffers many tiny abrasions during the friction of sex.

It is important to use the condom correctly. It should be rolled on only when the penis is erect, pressing out any air by rolling it down firmly and fully. After sex, your partner should withdraw quickly, holding on to the base of the condom as he does so, to prevent any leakage of semen.

It is still unfortunately true that very many heterosexual men – and women – are not keen on the condom, as it may spoil the spontaneity of lovemaking. But that is rather a secondary concern when there is the risk of AIDS. If women start to insist on condom use because of the risk, men are more likely to start adjusting to using them too. If they won't, it is probably worth giving those men a miss.

Anal sex, where there is any risk your partner may be carrying the HIV virus, should always be avoided. Ordinary condoms are not strong enough for this purpose. Swallowing semen is of uncertain wisdom. Semen carries a high concentration of the virus if the male is infected but may be destroyed by the gut before it can do damage elsewhere. To be on the safe side, it should be avoided.

Women contemplating artificial insemination by a donor should be aware that the virus has been passed on in this way and should check that donors are being screened first.

If you seriously think you may be at risk of having caught the virus because of your lifestyle and you would like to get pregnant, it is a very good idea to be tested for the presence of antibodies to the virus. It is very ill-advised at present to get pregnant if you are positive, as pregnancy further weakens the immune system.

Choose your time to visit a genito-urinary clinic for a test wisely, as it can take up to three months after infection for antibodies to show in the blood. A positive result is likely to be a devastating experience psychologically. Clinics should have AIDS counsellors who can talk through the ramifications with you.

The Terrence Higgins Trust, a charity set up to advise and support people with AIDS or the HIV virus, has a helpline you can ring any evening from 7-10 p.m. The number is 01-833 2971.

13.
HEPATITIS B

WHAT IS IT?

Hepatitis B is a viral infection which causes inflammation of the liver and can have potentially serious complications. In this country it is very commonly contracted sexually, which is why it is included here. It is about 100 times more infectious than AIDS (i.e. it is 100 times easier to catch it). Even after sufferers have recovered, some – usually men – become silent carriers of the disease and can pass it on for the rest of their lives. They are also more at risk of long-term complications themselves. One person in 1000 in Britain is probably a carrier.

WHAT ARE THE SYMPTOMS?

Symptoms are the same in men and women. It takes between one and three months after contact with the virus for any symptoms to appear at all and these are usually tiredness, loss of appetite and nausea. About half of the people who get hepatitis B have no more symptoms than these at all. Or else this stage may be followed by jaundice, fever, tenderness in the area of the liver and a tendency for urine to be darker than usual while stools are lighter. This acute illness phase may last up to a fortnight but be followed by a lengthy depression and lethargy, often for as long as six months.

HOW DO YOU GET IT?

The hepatitis B virus is commonly acquired by sex with a partner who is currently infected or a carrier of the disease. It is most usually blood-borne and enters the body through cuts and abrasions but can also be passed in semen and vaginal secretions. About 28 per cent of female partners of chronic carriers have antibodies to the disease. It is extremely common in homosexuals or bisexuals because anal intercourse usually causes bruising and bleeding.

Non-sexual methods of acquiring hepatitis B are mainly by splashes of contaminated blood entering through a cut in the skin or via needle pricks. Medical and nursing staff, dentists and hygienists are at high risk. So, of course, are intravenous drug users. More general sources of infection are contaminated needles not sterilised properly after use for acupuncture, ear piercing, tattooing and electrolysis.

WHAT ARE THE RISKS IF UNTREATED?

There hasn't been any effective treatment for hepatitis B (but see section on treatment below for new advances). The disease wears off on its own, slowly. However, if high levels of the virus remain present in the blood for more than six months, the person becomes a carrier. This happens in one in ten cases. Long term risks include relapses of the disease, cirrhosis and liver cancer – the risk of the latter for chronic carriers is 273 times that for non-carriers.

Babies can acquire hepatitis B from their mothers at or around the time of birth.

WHAT IS THE TREATMENT?

In trials in Holland, a drug combination of acyclovir and interferon has been found to produce regression in a significant number of chronic hepatitis sufferers and is being investigated further.

Vaccines are now available to protect at-risk groups from contracting hepatitis B. They are not 100 per cent effective, however, and only protect for a certain number of years.

HOW TO HELP YOURSELF

If you have bisexual partners, you are more at risk of contracting hepatitis. Use condoms and avoid anal intercourse and swallowing semen.

Women who have recently had hepatitis should avoid the contraceptive pill or be tested first to ensure their liver function is normal.

Check when having any commercial procedure that entails a needle prick, such as electrolysis, that the practitioner uses an autoclave for sterilisation or better still uses disposable needles.

14.
PLAYING
SAFE

By the law of averages, the more sexual partners you
have, the greater your chances of acquiring a sexually
transmitted disease. While that isn't always such a dire
fate, what is worrying nowadays is the number of women
who suffer long-term consequences, particularly
infertility or cervical cancer, because the disease they
caught did not kindly alert them to its presence with
symptoms and therefore had time to do its damage in
peace.

Into that category must also come the little-known
cytomegalovirus and Group-B streptococci, infections
which can be passed sexually as well as caught in other
ways. They rarely give rise to symptoms, but if present
when giving birth can cause serious abnormalities in a
baby.

A few years ago in America, when herpes hysteria was
in all the headlines, a great many women swore
themselves to celibacy thereafter. More have done so since
AIDS. What is important, however, is to make choices
about your own sexual life in the light of all the facts
and to be aware that it isn't just what you do that counts,
it is what your partner does too. If you choose to take
sexual risks, then at least be responsible about
minimising any consequences for yourself and for your
partner. It isn't enough to check first that a new passing

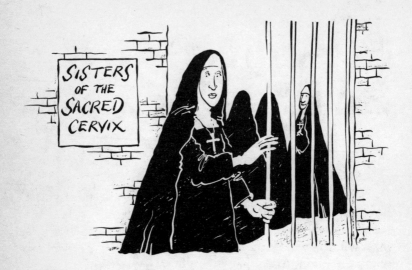

partner is all right on the night. Symptoms of sexually transmitted diseases can take time to show, by which time he might have gone off into the pale blue yonder.

Conversely, even if you have only ever had one partner and are still with him, do not be complacent unless you are absolutely positive that your partner is always faithful to you. And some unpleasant, although not dangerous, infections can of course be caught whether you have a sexual partner or not.

Here is a summary of all the main sensible precautions all women can take, regardless of their lifestyle, to minimise the risk of catching or harbouring undesirable alien organisms.

CHOICE OF CONTRACEPTION

Think carefully about your method of contraception. Barrier methods such as the condom and the diaphragm used particularly with a spermicide containing

Nonoxynol-9 make sense. Nonoxynol-9 appears to have happy protective effects against herpes, chlamydia, gonorrhoea and even AIDS, although undoubtedly it can never be foolproof. The contraceptive sponge, which like the condom is available from chemists without a prescription, also contains Nonoxynol-9.

However if you do have sex with more than one partner, regularly or occasionally, it is really most advisable to use a condom during the casual encounters, whatever your normal method of contraception. The condom is the only method which protects you from any contact with a partner's semen, vital in the prevention of AIDS, where the virus can enter the body through tiny abrasions in the skin caused by friction during sex.

The pill increases protection against gonorrhoea but reduces it against chlamydia. The IUD is definitely a bad idea for anyone who has several sexual partners, especially if they have never had children, as it increases susceptibility to infections, some of which may cause infertility.

VAGINAL CARE AND HYGIENE

Whatever your lifestyle, avoid an over-obsession with vaginal cleanliness. Don't ever use antiseptics around this delicate area and go for simple soaps rather than perfumed ones. Bubble baths and treats of this ilk should not be indulged in by anyone who is prone to thrush or cystitis. If you feel sore and itchy in the genital area, it may be because of chemicals in the bathroom cosmetics or it may be a sign of the presence of some infection. Whatever the cause, it is not advisable to put on soothing creams which may mask the symptoms and make the problem worse.

One form of hygiene it is important to be obsessive about, however, it not transferring germs from the rectum to the vagina or urethra. Never wipe yourself from back to front.

Avoid wearing trousers which are too tight – at least, don't do it too often – and don't put nylon next to your skin. You'll be creating a hothouse in which various germs can thrive.

If sometimes you don't lubricate properly when you are going to have sex – lubrication is affected by hormones and mood amongst other things – don't bash on regardless or you will bruise delicate tissue. Make use of a vaginal lubricant, as sold for the purpose in chemists.

CERVICAL SMEARS

If you are sexually active, you should have regular cervical smears taken, either from your doctor (if he or she will), your family planning clinic or a genito-urinary clinic. The standard recommendation is a smear once every five years, but if you have a history of sexually transmitted diseases, particularly herpes or genital warts, some experts think you should be tested once a year. You can but try – so ask for one. Always make sure you *get the result*. Ring yourself to be sure, even if you are assured that you will be contacted if the smear is positive. Errors can happen.

DIET

Make sure you have a good diet. Good nutrition nowadays is often vaunted as the answer to all ills. Whether that is entirely true or not, don't knock it. A diet that is plentiful in fresh fruits and vegetables will contain the vitamins and minerals that help the body's immune system to perform at peak level and resist far more infections.

GENITO-URINARY CLINICS

If you do have several sexual partners, or if you know
your partner does, go to a genito-urinary clinic for a check-
up at least once a year just to be on the safe side. Always
go if you notice any symptoms of any kind – but wait
till a few days after their first appearance so that any
infection will show up for certain on examination.

I have recommended several times in this book that
the genito-urinary clinic should be the first choice, rather
than your doctor's surgery, for the investigation of any
possible genito-urinary infection. The doctors here are
the experts and they deal with a whole range of problems
from sexually transmitted diseases, vaginal and bladder
infections through to problems with sex or with
contraception. They are very different places from the
old 'special' or VD clinics and their image has changed
accordingly.

You do not need to be referred to one by your doctor
and what goes on in the clinic remains between you and
the clinic. Some operate appointment systems – you
simply ring up and make one – others see you in order
of your arrival on any day. The advantage of the
appointment system is that you do not have to spend so
long on the premises waiting to be seen, although it may
take a week before you get an appointment. The
advantage of the drop-in system is that, although it takes
longer, you will be seen that day.

Staff at genito-urinary clinics go out of their way to
be relaxed and confidence-inspiring. They are not stern
judgmental individuals who will subject all who sit before
them to a lecture on clean living, especially as a great
many of their patients don't require it. They are only
interested in your health. To this end, however, they will
ask a lot of questions, from the date of your last period
to when you last had sex and whether you have had any
other partners in the last few months. They will ask these

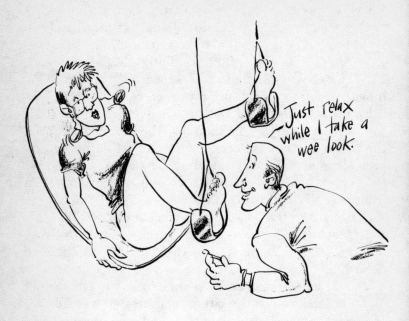

questions even if you are attending just because you think
you have thrush and it is nothing to be embarrassed
about. You should mention anything that has crossed
your mind as possibly vaguely relevant, even if you think
it might sound a bit silly. All symptoms will be taken
seriously and you won't get laughed at. Always tell the
doctor if you are pregnant or trying to become pregnant,
as this may affect which drugs are used for your
treatment.

The consultation is followed by an internal
examination. Many women dislike internals and
consequently tense their muscles, which makes the whole
process more uncomfortable. If you can allow yourself
to relax, it is usually painless. The doctor will feel for
any tenderness or inflammation inside and out. Usually
he or she will do this after taking samples from cells for

116

testing. To do this, he or she will insert a speculum in the vagina to hold the walls open – again, usually painless if you can relax – and gently take samples or scrapings from any or all of the vagina, the cervix, the urethra and the rectum. The feeling is one of a prinprick, if that, and it takes just a second.

You may also be asked at some point for a urine sample and, almost always, some blood will be taken for testing. All this enables laboratory staff to test for a wide variety of infections. Whatever your symptoms or the concern which brought you, they will test for thrush, trichomonas, gonorrhoea and syphilis. Usually they will test for gardnerella and in more and more clinics, they will also test for chlamydia. Tests for herpes are only done if signs are present or if your partner has herpes. Any warts that are spotted will be treated during the genital examination.

After all this is over, you return to the waiting room for how ever long it takes for the samples to be looked at down a microscope – it could be ten minutes, it could be an hour, depending on the queue. Some results will be available instantly and any necessary treatment can be started. For others, tests need to be carried out in a laboratory and for these you have to return in a week or so – having abstained from sex in the interim. It is very important to go back on the day you are told to, so that treatment can start, if any is needed.

If you do have anything which can be sexually transmitted, it is vital to tell your partner to go to the clinic for treatment too. For some infections, the doctor who sees you may provide you with tablets for you both. It is very important to be honest about how many partners may have been infected.

It can, of course, be a shock to learn that you have a particular infection. If you have been living a monogamous life, you may be puzzled, upset or plain angry. You may have certain unconscious beliefs about the 'type of person' who gets such diseases. There is no such person – whoever is sexually active is to some degree at risk. Or, if it is something like herpes or genital warts which can come back at any time, you may feel anxious or uncertain how to cope. Usually in genito-urinary clinics there is someone skilled in counselling who you can ask to see and talk to about the realities rather than the myths, usually putting your mind at rest. Things we read in the media tend to be more doom-laden and dire than the true circumstances warrant. The counsellors can also provide advice and a listening ear if you need to talk over how to involve your partner or how you feel about the effect of an infection on your relationship.

But forewarned is forearmed. I hope this book has helped.

ABOUT THE AUTHOR

DENISE WINN is a freelance writer and journalist specializing in medical and psychological topics.

A former editor of *Psychology Today* and of the magazine produced by MIND (National Association for Mental Health), she is the medical writer for *Cosmopolitan* and contributes regularly to other magazines and newspapers.

She has written seven books. *The Hospice Way*, about the special quality of care offered by hospices to the terminally ill, is also published by Optima.

More books from Optima . . .

FRIENDS OF THE EARTH HANDBOOK

edited by Jonathon Porritt

A great many people are interested in protecting the environment, but are not sure what they should do about it. This is a practical guide on how to put environmental ideals into practice.

Topics discussed include the best ways to save energy, waste disposal, the use of water, transport policies, the protection of wildlife and the politics of food.

ISBN 0 356 12560 2

Price (in UK only) **£4.95**

THE HOSPICE WAY by Denise Winn

Public interest in hospices and the care of the terminally ill is growing.

Denise Winn explains in a sympathetic way what hospice care means, the aims and philosophy of hospices, and how these are put into effect, including the control of pain, the underlying acceptance of death, and the welcome extended to patients' families and friends.

Advice is given on how to find a hospice and at what stage, any financial arrangements, and the possibility of hospice-style care at home.

ISBN 0 356 12741 9

Price (in UK only) **£3.95**

YOUR BRILLIANT CAREER by Audrey Slaughter

This handbook by Audrey Slaughter, well-known Fleet Street editor, offers a wealth of very practical advice for women of all ages on how to turn a job into a career, with information about training and specific management skills, as well as a self-confidence and mental attitude.

The book includes useful hints from women at the top, and will be of real help to all working women.

ISBN 0 356 12705 2

Price (in UK only) **£4.95**

STONE AGE DIET by Leon Chaitow
Leon Chaitow, well-known nutritionist and author, explores
the idea that the diet of our Stone Age ancestors was not only
healthy, enabling them to develop the most stable society
known in world history, but also very much in keeping with
modern nutritional advice.

The book is firmly based on the latest scientific research,
and includes a number of appropriate recipes.
ISBN 0 356 12328 6
Price (in UK only) **£4.95**

SELF HELP WITH PMS by Dr Michelle Harrison
One of the most comprehensive books available on the subject
of PMS (premenstrual syndrome), it covers *all* its symptoms,
both physical and mental, including the much publicized topic
of premenstrual tension. The forms of treatment are fully
described in clear, everyday language. Case histories and up-to-
date details of new research into treatment are also
included.

Illustrated with humorous but sympathetic line drawings,
this book is an indispensable guide for the large number of
women who suffer from this syndrome every month.
ISBN 0 356 12559 9
Price (in UK only) **£5.95**

MENOPAUSE THE NATURAL WAY
by Dr Sadja Greenwood
A compehensive book that answers all the questions a woman
could possibly ask about the menopause. Myths about the
menopause are corrected and all medical details are clearly
explained in language that anyone can understand. All forms
of treatment for the problems associated with the menopause
are discussed, including the most up-to-date and controversial.
Includes case histories and is illustrated with humorous but
sympathetic line drawings, that complement the positive
approach of the book.

It will be welcomed by every woman (and a lot of men) as
a complete, practical guide to promoting good health and
avoiding illness in the second half of life.
ISBN 0 356 12561 0
Price (in UK only) **£5.95**

ALTERNATIVE HEALTH SERIES

This series is designed to provide factual information and practical advice about alternative therapies. While including essential details of theory and history, the books concentrate on what patients can expect during treatment, how they should prepare for it, what questions will be asked and why, what form the treatment will take, what it will 'feel' like and how soon they can expect to respond.

1. ACUPUNCTURE by Michael Nightingale
   Acupuncture is a traditional Chinese therapy which usually (but not always) uses needles to stimulate the body's own energy and so bring healing.
   ISBN 0 356 12426 6
   Price (in UK only) **£3.95**

2. OSTEOPATHY by Stephen Sandler
   Osteopathy started in the USA in the 1870s, and has since spread to many other countries. It is a manipulative therapy, where the osteopath heals by adjusting the position of bones and tissues.
   ISBN 0 356 12428 2
   Price (in UK only) **£3.95**

DOWN TO EARTH – A CALENDAR FOR THE RELUCANT GARDENER by Mike Gillian with Alan Titchmarsh

DOWN TO EARTH, like the associated radio programme, is for every gardener who only wants to potter for a couple of hours at the weekend, and still expects results. There's one main, illustrated job for each week, plus topical tips on smaller 'odd jobs'. The style is lively, the approach not always orthodox, and subjects range widely – lawns, hedges, flowers, ponds, trees, even discouraging unwelcome cats. The emphasis is on the easy, instant results and maximum effect for minimum cost and effort.
ISBN 0 356 12704 4
Price (in UK only) **£4.95**

All Optima books are available at your bookshop or newsagent, or can be ordered from the following address:

Optima, Cash Sales Department,
P.O. Box 11, Falmouth, Cornwall.

Please send cheque or postal order (no currency), and allow 55p for postage and packing for the first book plus 22p for the second book and 14p for each additional book ordered up to a maxdimum charge of £1.75 in U.K.

Customers in Eire and B.F.P.O. please allow 55p for the first book, 22p for the second book plus 14p per copy for the next 7 books, thereafter 8p per book.

Overseas customers please allow £1 for postage and packing for the first book and 25p per copy for each additional book.